LEADER'S MANUAL FOR ADOLESCENT GROUPS

LEADER'S MANUAL FOR ADOLESCENT GROUPS

ADOLESCENT COPING WITH DEPRESSION COURSE

Gregory Clarke, Ph.D.
Peter Lewinsohn, Ph.D.
Hyman Hops, Ph.D.

With consultation from Bonnie Grossen, Ph.D.

Castalia Publishing Company
P.O. Box 1587
Eugene, OR 97440

ISBN 0-916154-20-3
Printed in the United States of America

Copies of this manual may be ordered from the publisher.

Editorial and Production Credits
        Editor-in-Chief: Scot G. Patterson
        Associate Editor: Margo Moore
        Copy Editor: Ruth Cornell
        Cover Design: Astrografix
        Page Composition: Margo Moore

CONTENTS

DEDICATION

To the adolescents, families, and colleagues who have helped us over the years to develop this treatment program for depression.

ACKNOWLEDGEMENTS

Many talented people have contributed to the development of the Adolescent Coping with Depression Course. Foremost among these was Ms. Bonnie Grossen, whose many valuable suggestions have made the course more "teachable." The manuals also reflect the efforts of the therapists who helped to pilot and critique the preliminary and current versions of the course: Paul Rohde, Michael Horn, Jackie Bianconi, Carolyn Alexander, Patricia DeGroot, Kathryn Frye, Gail Getz, Kathleen Hennig, Richard Langford, Karen Lloyd, Pat Neil-Carlton, Margie Myska, Mary Pederson, Evelyn Schenk, Ned Duncan, Julie Williams, Julie Redner, Beth Blackshaw, Karen Poulin, Kathy Vannatta, Johannes Rothlind, Galyn Forster, Nancy Winters, Scott Fisher, Renee Marcy, Susan Taylor, and Shirley Hanson.

We would also like to acknowledge that the concepts and techniques presented in the course reflect the work of the following authors and researchers (among others): Aaron Beck, M.D., Albert Ellis, Ph.D., Marion Forgatch, Ph.D., Susan Glaser, Ph.D., John Gottman, Ph.D., Gerald Kranzler, Ph.D., Lenore Radloff, M.S., Arthur Robin, Ph.D., and Irvin Yalom, M.D.

Our sincere thanks to Scot Patterson and Margo Moore for their persistence and expertise in editing and preparing this manual for publication; their assistance has been invaluable.

PREFACE

This book describes the cognitive-behavioral treatment program that has been developed by our research team for adolescent unipolar depression. The treatment is conducted with groups of four to eight participants who are 14 to 18 years of age, and the vehicle for therapy is a class entitled the "Adolescent Coping with Depression Course." During the sixteen 2-hour sessions, the adolescents learn essential skills for overcoming depression. The areas covered are relaxation, pleasant events, irrational and negative thoughts, social skills, communication, and problem solving. Several different methods of instruction are employed: lectures by the group leader, discussions, role-playing exercises, and homework assignments. Research on the efficacy of the treatment program has demonstrated that more than 70% of the adolescents who have participated in the course are significantly improved one month after termination, and that these gains are maintained up to 12 months after treatment.

Depression is a debilitating disorder that seriously affects the lives of hundreds of thousands of teenagers in the United States. Bouts of clinical depression also place the adolescent at risk for a number of associated problems such as academic difficulties and suicide. In addition, social withdrawal and the other obstacles to social functioning that often accompany the disorder have a dramatic impact on many aspects of the adolescent's life at a critical time in his or her development. Although episodes of clinical depression may gradually subside, the likelihood that these episodes and/or depressive symptoms will recur is extremely high unless there is some kind of intervention.

Until recently, depression among adolescents has received very little attention, and there have been few treatment resources available other than traditional psychotherapy and medication. The Adolescent Coping with Depression Course is a cost-effective, nonstigmatizing, psychoeducational intervention that can be used in a variety of clinical settings such as schools, mental health centers, and hospitals. It is our hope that the course will help to meet the need for an effective treatment program that is specifically designed for use with adolescents.

INTRODUCTION

It is only during the last two decades that adolescent depression has become the focus of public and scientific interest. Previously, depression was considered to be extremely rare or even nonexistent in children and teenagers (see review by Carlson and Garber, 1986). In recent years, however, several large-scale epidemiological studies have shown that clinical depression among teenagers is a significant problem, affecting up to 3% of the general high school population at any one point in time (Kashani, Holcomb, and Orvaschel, 1986; Lewinsohn, Hops, Roberts, and Seeley, 1988). By age 18, up to 20% of all teenagers have had at least one episode of clinical depression (Lewinsohn et al., 1988). These rates make depression *the most frequently reported mental health problem for this age group.*

Early studies significantly advanced the nosology of affective disorders in children and adolescents (Orvaschel and Puig-Antich, 1986; Friedman, Hurt, Clarkin, Corn, and Aronoff, 1983; Chambers, Puig-Antich, Hirsch, Paez, Ambrosini, Tabrizi, and Davies, 1985). These and other studies have contributed to the present consensus that the central symptoms of adolescent depression are similar, if not identical, to those of adult affective disorders (Kazdin, Sherick, Esveldt-Dawson, and Rancurello, 1985; Strauss, Forehand, Frame, and Smith, 1984; Seligman, Peterson, Kaslow, Tanenbaum, Alloy, and Abramson, 1984).

Unfortunately, recent evidence suggests that the prevalence of depression has been on the rise among adolescents (Klerman and Weissman, 1989). For example, over the past two decades there has been a *200% to 400% increase* in the number of teenage suicides across the United States (Shaffer and Fisher, 1981), which indicates there has been a similar increase in the rates of depressive disorder. Still other studies suggest a link between teenage drug/alcohol abuse, suicide, and depression (Lewinsohn, Hops, Roberts, and Seeley, 1988; Kandel and Davies, 1982). Certainly, the likelihood of other coexisting disorders is markedly elevated in adolescents who have had an episode of affective disorder (Lewinsohn, Hops, Roberts, and Seeley, 1988). It is clear that depression among adolescents is a major mental health problem, with numerous negative sequela and associated difficulties.

Treatment of Adolescent Depression

In contrast to these advances in diagnosis and nosology, there have been relatively few investigations to date of the psychotherapeutic treatment of adolescent depression. Until recently, published accounts of the treatment of child and adolescent depression consisted exclusively of single case studies (Petti, Bornstein, Delemeter, and Conners, 1980; Frame, Matson, Sonis, Falkov, and Kazdin, 1982). During the last several years, a few investigators have initiated larger experimental studies of psychological group treatments for depression in adolescents and children.

Butler et al. (1980) focused on the school-based identification and treatment of depressed children 10 to 13 years of age. Several different interventions were compared: 1) Role Play, which emphasized social skills and problem solving; 2) Cognitive Restructuring, which focused on the identification and modification of automatic and self-deprecating thoughts; 3) a teacher mediated attention-placebo control group; and 4) a classroom control group, which was never assigned to any intervention. Children in the Role Play group demonstrated the greatest decline in self-reported depression, while the children in the Cognitive Restructuring group showed evidence of a minor but nonsignificant trend toward improvement. Children in the two control conditions failed to exhibit any significant improvement.

Reynolds and Coats (1986) randomly assigned 30 adolescents with elevated scores on the Beck Depression Inventory (Beck et al., 1961) to one of three conditions: a cognitive-behavioral treatment program, relaxation training, or a waiting-list control group. The two treatment approaches were highly structured and involved homework assignments and self-monitoring. Each treatment consisted of ten 50-minute sessions conducted over a 5-week period. Subjects in both active treatments showed substantial and equal improvement; subjects in the waiting-list control group did not change significantly between pre-treatment, post-treatment, and follow-up assessments.

While the results of these studies are encouraging, both the Butler et al. (1980) and Reynolds and Coats (1986) studies relied on self-report measures such as the Beck Depression Inventory or the Child Depression Inventory to *define* their cases of "depression" (cases which may or may not have met DSM-III-R criteria for clinical depression). In addition, each study employed these same self-report measures as the *primary indication of treatment outcome*. Conclusions regarding outcome were based solely on patient self-report, which is often subject to various response biases. Expert clinical judgment, which is presumably less subject to error, was not included. At the very least, multiple perspectives (e.g., parent, child, clinician, and teacher) should be employed in evaluating outcome.

Despite these shortcomings, the positive results of these studies are encouraging and suggest that the cognitive-behavioral techniques originally developed for use with depressed adults can be successfully adapted for use with adolescents and children in a group format.

The Adolescent Coping With Depression Course

The Adolescent Coping with Depression Course is a psychoeducational, cognitive-behavioral intervention for adolescent depression. The course is closely modeled after the adult Coping with Depression Course (Lewinsohn,

Antonuccio, Steinmetz-Breckenridge, and Teri, 1984). While the adolescent course is very similar to the adult treatment program, the content has been modified and simplified. The lectures and homework assignments have been reduced, and there is greater emphasis on group activities and role-playing exercises. An earlier version of the course (Clarke and Lewinsohn, 1986) consisted of fourteen 2-hour sessions which were held twice each week for seven weeks; the current version (Clarke, Lewinsohn, and Hops, 1990) consists of sixteen 2-hour sessions conducted over an 8-week period.

The course is designed for use with groups of four to eight adolescents as an after-school program and in other settings, or it can be modified for use on an individual basis. The treatment sessions are conducted as a class in which a group leader teaches adolescents skills for controlling depression. The areas covered include relaxation, pleasant events, negative thoughts, social skills, communication, and problem solving. Each adolescent is provided with a *Student Workbook* which is closely integrated with course discussions and group activities. The workbook contains brief readings, structured learning tasks, self-monitoring forms, homework assignments, and short quizzes.

The parents of the adolescents are encouraged to participate in the program to help foster and maintain positive changes in the adolescents' moods. The course for parents consists of nine 2-hour sessions that are held once each week on one of the same nights as the adolescent group. During these sessions, parents are given an overview of the skills and techniques that are taught to their adolescents. This promotes parental acceptance and reinforcement of the positive changes in their teenagers. Most of the sessions for parents and adolescents are separate, with the exception of two sessions in which they practice problem-solving and negotiation skills as a family. Detailed guidelines for running the parent groups are provided in a leader's manual by Lewinsohn, Rohde, Hops, and Clarke (1990); a workbook for parents is also available.

An important feature of the course is that it is nonstigmatizing because the treatment is presented and conducted as a class and not as therapy. It is a cost-effective, community-oriented approach that can successfully reach the great majority of depressed adolescents who typically do not make use of the services of school counselors, therapists, and other mental health professionals.

The Course Sessions

The course is presented as an opportunity for adolescents to learn new skills which will help them to gain control over their moods and deal with situations that contribute to their depression. During the first session, the group leader reviews the rules and guidelines for the course, the underlying rationale, and the social learning view of depression. The remaining sessions focus on teaching specific skills (relaxation, pleasant activities, constructive thinking, social skills, communication, and negotiation and problem solving). Figure 1 provides a summary of the skill areas that are covered during each session.

Specific Skill	**Figure 1: Timeline of Skills and Sessions** Session															
	1	2	3	4	5	6	7	8	9	10	11	12	13	14	15	16
Mood Monitoring	■	░	░	░	░	░	░	░	░	░	░	░	░	░	░	░
Social Skills	■	■	■	■	■	■	■	■		░						░
Pleasant Activities		■	░	■	■	░	░	░	░	░	░	░			░	░
Relaxation			■	░	░	░	░	■	░	░	░	░	░			░
Constructive Thinking					■	■	■	■	■	■						░
Communication									■	■	■	■	░	░		░
Negotiation and Problem Solving											■	■	■	■		░
Maintaining Gains															■	■

Key

■■■■ = Skill is taught

░░░░ = Skill is discussed as part of home practice

Relaxation Sessions

The first relaxation technique presented is the Jacobsen method, in which participants alternately tense and relax major muscle groups throughout the body until they are fully relaxed (Jacobsen, 1929). This relaxation technique is introduced early in the course because it is relatively easy to learn and it provides the adolescents with an initial success experience; it is thought that this enhances their sense of perceived self-efficacy (Bandura, 1981), which has been hypothesized to be a critical component of successful psychotherapeutic interventions (Zeiss, Lewinsohn, and Muñoz, 1979). The Benson method is introduced about mid-way through the course; this relaxation technique involves sitting comfortably in a quiet place and repeating a word or phrase. Adolescents also learn a variation called the "quick" Benson that is more portable than the Jacobsen technique.

Another rationale for including relaxation training is the well-demonstrated correlation and co-morbidity between depression and anxiety (Maser and Clonniger, 1989), and the related hypothesis that depression and anxiety may be etiologically related disorders. If there is a causal relationship, providing treatment for anxiety would assist adolescents in their recovery from depression.

Many depressed adolescents also report experiencing tension and anxiety during social events and in other stressful situations. This anxiety often interferes with effective interpersonal functioning and reduces the pleasure derived from potentially enjoyable activities. Teaching depressed adolescents to relax in situations that are typically stressful enables them to implement the social skills they learn during the course and enjoy pleasant activities more (many of which are socially-oriented).

Pleasant Activities Sessions

The rationale for including sessions that focus on pleasant activities is based on the behavioral theory of depression developed by Lewinsohn and his colleagues (Lewinsohn, Biglan, and Zeiss, 1976). The primary hypothesis of this behavioral formulation is that relatively low rates of response-contingent positive reinforcement (positive social interactions, pleasant activities, etc.) are a critical antecedent for the occurrence of unipolar depression. This hypothesis emphasizes the importance of helping depressed individuals increase their levels of pleasant activities, while at the same time decreasing their levels of negative or punishing events.

Adolescents learn several basic self-change skills during the pleasant activities sessions. These skills include monitoring specific behaviors that have been targeted for change, establishing a baseline, setting realistic goals, and developing a plan and a contract for making changes in their behavior. Activities for each adolescent to increase are identified through the use of the Pleasant Events Schedule (PES) developed by MacPhillamy and Lewinsohn (1982). The PES contains a list of 320 potentially pleasant activities (e.g., "Taking a walk," and "Reading a book"). An adolescent version of the PES is included in the appendix of the *Student Workbook*. To fill out the schedule, each adolescent must go through the list twice. First, the adolescent rates each event according to how often it occurred during the past 30 days; the second time through the list, each event is rated for its actual or potential enjoyability. When the PES is scored, an individualized list of pleasant activities is generated for each adolescent (*note:* a computerized scoring program for the PES is available from the publisher).

Cognitive Therapy Sessions

The cognitive therapy sessions address the negative and irrational thoughts known to be associated with depression in adolescents. The approach is based on the theories of Beck (e.g., Beck, Rush, Shaw, and Emery, 1979) and Ellis (e.g., Ellis and Harper, 1961), which hypothesize that depression is both caused and maintained by negative or irrational beliefs. The sessions incorporate elements of the interventions developed by Beck et al. (1979) and Ellis and Harper (1961) for identifying and challenging negative and irrational thoughts, although these techniques have been modified and simplified for use with adolescents. For example, cartoon strips with popular characters (Garfield, Bloom County, etc.) are employed to illustrate negative thinking and the use of positive counterthoughts to dispute irrational beliefs. Through a series of progressively more advanced exercises, adolescents learn how to apply cognitive techniques to their own personal thoughts.

Social Skills Sessions

Several studies have demonstrated that depression is highly associated with poor social functioning, both in adults (e.g., Lewinsohn, Mischel, Chaplin, and Barton, 1980; Weissman and Paykel, 1974) and adolescents (e.g., Puig-Antich, Lukens, Davies, Goetz, Brennan-Quattrock, and Todak, 1985). This lack of social skills may contribute to the onset of depressive episodes, and may also be involved in maintaining and prolonging them. To address these deficits, the social skills sessions give adolescents opportunities to learn and practice a variety of techniques such as active listening, planning social activities, and strategies for making friends. In contrast to the other content areas, the social skills sessions are interspersed throughout the course (see Figure 1), to ensure that they are integrated with the other techniques and skills taught in the class (especially relaxation and pleasant activities).

Communication, Negotiation, and Problem-Solving Sessions

A unique aspect of the course is its focus on basic communication, negotiation, and conflict resolution skills (Sessions 9 through 14). The rationale for including these techniques is based on the hypothesis that familial conflict escalates as teenagers progressively assert their independence, and that the inability to resolve issues leads to negative interactions which may in turn contribute to or maintain the adolescent's depression. The specific negotiation and communication techniques employed in the course are based on the ideas developed by Robin (Robin, 1977, 1979; Robin, Kent, O'Leary, Foster, and Prinz, 1977), Gottman (Gottman, Notarius, Gonso, and Markman, 1976), and Forgatch (Forgatch and Patterson, 1989), which emphasize the importance of good communication skills for effective problem solving (Alexander, 1973; Alexander, Barton, Schiavo, and Parsons, 1976; Robin and Weiss, 1980).

The problem-solving sessions use a four-step model, based on Robin's (1979, 1981) approach: 1) define the problem concisely and without accusations, 2) brainstorm alternative solutions, 3) decide on a mutually satisfactory solution through a structured negotiation process, and 4) specify the details for implementing the agreement.

The communication training involves feedback, modeling, and behavior rehearsal to correct negative behaviors such as accusations, interruptions, partial listening, lectures, and put-downs. These are replaced with positive behaviors such as paraphrasing, active listening, "I" messages, good eye contact, and appropriate body language.

Life Plan and Maintaining Gains Sessions

The last two sessions focus on integrating the skills that have been learned, anticipating future problems, maintaining therapy gains, developing a Life Plan and associated goals, and preventing relapses. Participants also identify the skills that they have found to be most effective for controlling their moods. With the help of the group leader, each adolescent develops an "emergency plan" which describes the steps that will be taken to prevent depression in the future.

SECTION I
Background and Overview

The first section of this manual contains eight chapters that provide essential information regarding the theoretical and practical considerations related to conducting the Adolescent Coping with Depression Course. Mental health professionals who are preparing to offer the course in other settings should read these chapters carefully. There are many issues involved in working with adolescent depression that are critical to the success or failure of the program and the welfare of course participants. Many of these important issues are examined in this section.

Chapter 1 reviews the minimum qualifications for group leaders and the training models used in our research program. The instruments and procedures for the assessment of clinical depression and associated problems are described in Chapter 2. The focus of Chapter 3 is on strategies for recruiting participants, and inclusion and exclusion criteria. Chapter 4 considers some of the issues involved in conducting groups, such as fostering cohesiveness, developing trust and rapport, and dealing with attendance problems. Various possible adaptations of the course are discussed in Chapter 5. In Chapter 6, the theoretical foundation of the course and clinical implications are examined. Chapter 7 summarizes the research studies on the efficacy of the Coping with Depression Course as a treatment program for adults and adolescents. Goals for future research are outlined in Chapter 8.

CHAPTER 1
Selecting and Training Group Leaders

Our research group has trained numerous instructors to lead groups for adolescents and parents during the three outcome studies that have been conducted. Because our program was designed as a research investigation, we have developed strict recruitment criteria and training goals for our staff. Some of these criteria may not be appropriate in other settings such as clinics, private practices, and school counseling offices. Nonetheless, these criteria and goals will be reviewed here to identify significant training issues that should be considered by other mental health professionals who are using these materials. We believe that the success of our treatment program is due in part to the effort we have put into carefully selecting and training instructors, and that care providers in other settings will benefit from our experience.

Qualifications for Group Leaders

Group leaders must have a certain amount of relevant experience and training before attempting to offer the course. The purpose of specifying the minimum qualifications that we believe are necessary to lead groups is to ensure that the course is conducted in a therapeutically responsible and effective manner. A broad range of mental health professionals would have the necessary skills, assuming they have had some training in the assessment and treatment of adolescent affective and nonaffective disorders. The list includes psychologists, psychiatrists, psychiatric social workers and psychiatric nurse practitioners, and counselors. Individuals who are not adequately trained for independent practice (e.g., students, and teachers who do not have a mental health background) should only conduct the course under the supervision of a licensed mental health professional.

Adolescents enrolled in the course regularly present many challenges beyond those addressed in the *Leader's Manual*. Many issues that are critical to the success of the intervention are not covered, such as suicide risk assessment, group dynamics, and normal adolescent development. It is important for group leaders to have supervised training and/or experience in the following areas:

1. Crisis assessment and intervention, especially with suicidal and/or substance-abusive youth (see Pfeffer, 1986; Rotheram, 1987; Trautman and Shaffer, 1984).
2. Assessment of affective *and* nonaffective disorders (e.g., DSM-III-R). Group leaders must be able to identify adolescents who would *not* benefit from the treatment program (exclusion criteria are described in detail in Chapter 3).

3. Basic or intermediate training in any of the various cognitive-behavioral therapies, such as cognitive therapy (Beck, Rush, Shaw, and Emory, 1979; Burns, 1980), self-control therapy (Rehm, 1977), or Rational-Emotive Therapy (Ellis and Harper, 1961).
4. Experience leading psychotherapeutic groups, especially with adolescents and/or children.
5. Familiarity with basic relaxation techniques (e.g., Jacobsen, 1929).
6. Experience using behavioral techniques to manage conduct problems in adolescents and/or children.
7. A developmental perspective regarding the cognitive and emotional changes that take place during adolescence (particularly for adolescents 14 to 18 years old).
8. Familiarity with the social learning formulation of depressive disorders (Lewinsohn, Antonuccio, Steinmetz-Breckenridge, and Teri, 1984; Clarke and Lewinsohn, 1989).

Training Requirements

The *Leader's Manual* is very detailed and provides scripted lesson plans for each session. The *Student Workbook* is also very explicit and is well integrated with the lesson plans in the *Leader's Manual*. Nonetheless, therapists should not attempt to lead the course without some practice and/or supervised training. Because so much material is covered in each 2-hour session, leaders need to acquire hands-on familiarity with the manual in order to complete all of the lectures, tasks, and exercises in the time allowed. The first time leaders conduct the course, they are often so overwhelmed by the material in the lesson plans that they find it difficult to track both the *content* of the course as well as the important *clinical and process issues* that come up during the sessions.

Recommended Training Models

Of the several different models we have used to train new therapists, two approaches seem to work best. In the first model, a trainee therapist is paired with an experienced leader as a co-leader of the course. In the beginning, the experienced leader takes more responsibility for running the sessions, while the trainee therapist primarily observes. As the course progresses, however, the responsibility for conducting the sessions shifts as the trainee begins to take an increasingly active role. After each session, the experienced leader reviews the performance of the trainee and discusses possible solutions to the different clinical issues encountered during the session. Sometimes the sessions are videotaped so that the performance of the trainee can be examined in more detail. At the conclusion of the course, the trainee generally is ready to lead the course independently, provided that some supervision is available.

In the second training model, a "mock" course is conducted. An experienced therapist leads the group, and up to eight trainees assume the roles of adolescent participants. Each session is conducted in a start-stop manner to allow some additional time to review the rationale for specific aspects of the course, and to discuss problems or issues that commonly arise at different places in the sessions. After the first two or three sessions have been conducted in this manner by the experienced therapist, the trainees take turns running the group. Each trainee leads a minimum of two or more entire sessions. The experienced leader continues to interrupt sessions when necessary to discuss key issues or to clarify certain points. Group feedback is provided to trainee leaders after each session; the purpose of this feedback is to identify positive aspects of the trainee's performance and aspects that could be improved.

We have found that there are advantages and disadvantages to each of these training methods. The co-leader method offers direct experience with adolescent participants and gives each trainee an opportunity to lead more supervised sessions. However, the quality of the training is almost entirely dependent on the ability of the experienced therapist who supervises the sessions. If the experienced leader misunderstands or misapplies aspects of the intervention, it is likely that the trainee will use the same faulty methods. Another disadvantage to this training model is that it only permits the training of one new leader at a time.

In contrast, the mock group has regular, in-session discussions of the protocol, which makes misinterpretations of the intervention less likely. The larger number of trainees also means there is more variety in the opinions and solutions that are offered during discussions of problem issues. Another obvious advantage to this model is that several new leaders can be trained at one time. The major drawback to this approach is that it does not provide any experience working with adolescent participants.

From the discussion above, it seems evident that the ideal situation would be to have trainees begin by participating in a mock therapy group and then co-lead a course with an experienced leader (that is, the second training method followed by the first). In reality, trainees will probably be exposed to only one of these approaches. Thus, it is important to provide regular (weekly or bi-weekly) supervision for new therapists to discuss the therapeutic issues the are not explicitly addressed in the *Leader's Manual*.

CHAPTER 2
Assessment of Depression and Associated Problems

This chapter briefly reviews measures that are used in the assessment of clinical depression and depressive symptoms in adolescents, as well as instruments for assessing variables that have been shown to be related to depression. A more detailed review is available in Kaslow and Rehm (1985), and Kazdin (1987, 1988). The instruments discussed in this chapter will be considered primarily from a clinical perspective.

Until recently, there has been little research on childhood and adolescent depression, and there has also been a shortage of well-developed instruments with good psychometric properties. As pointed out in the Introduction, this lack of interest was due to a widespread belief that depression was not a problem for this population. During the last decade, however, research has demonstrated that the prevalence rates for depression among adolescents 14 to 18 years of age are similar to those for adults (Lewinsohn, Hops, Roberts, and Seeley, 1989). These results have served as an impetus for the development of multiple methods for assessing the depressive syndrome, its basic symptoms, and many of the related psychosocial constructs among adolescents.

For most purposes, assessment instruments can be divided into two categories: instruments that have been developed for clinical decision-making, and instruments that focus on research issues (see Lewinsohn and Rohde, 1987). There are three primary goals for clinical assessment: 1) to identify depressed or dysphoric adolescents in need of treatment, 2) to determine the specific deficits that preclude the adolescent's successful functioning (i.e., the targets for intervention that determine the specific treatment procedures), and 3) to evaluate the short-term and long-term impact of treatment. The goals for research assessment focus more on the clarification of theoretical issues, such as discriminating between different forms of affective disorders (e.g., unipolar vs. bipolar), comparing treatment procedures, and developing assessment instruments that provide data relevant to these goals. In general, clinical instruments need to be more cost-effective, easy to administer, adequately normed, and useful for practitioners. In research, with the exception of norms, these issues are less pertinent.

Self-report scales are the most commonly used instruments in clinical settings. Many of the fundamental symptoms of depressive disorders such as sadness and feelings of worthlessness are subjective, thus self-report plays an important role in the assessment of depression. The evidence suggests that adolescents are in the best position to report on their own feelings and behavior, although information from parents, teachers, and peers should be used to substantiate and supplement their self-report data.

Self-Report of Depressive Symptoms

Interviews

Although the primary objective of a clinical diagnostic interview is to determine whether an adolescent meets DSM-III-R criteria for Major Depressive Disorder or Dysthymia, the interview also generates clinically useful information. During the interview, the therapist can observe the behavior of the adolescents, which can be very important if they are reluctant to admit specific symptoms, have poor communication skills, or resist treatment. The diagnostic interview is a relatively systematic procedure for identifying the specific difficulties that the adolescent is experiencing.

There are at least three interviews that have been standardized for this purpose: The Schedule for Affective Disorders and Schizophrenia for School-Aged Children (K-SADS; Chambers, Puig-Antich, Hirsch, Paez, Ambrosini, Tabrizi, and Davies, 1985), the Diagnostic Interview for Children and Adolescents (DICA; Herjanich and Reich, 1982), and the Diagnostic Interview Schedule for Children (DISC; Costello, Edelbrock, and Costello, 1985). The K-SADS, which is an adaptation of the original adult version (Endicott and Spitzer, 1978), is probably the one most frequently used in clinical and research settings. The K-SADS interviews must be conducted by trained therapists with extensive clinical experience. The K-SADS begins with an unstructured interview; this is followed by a semi-structured interview in which the adolescent is asked about the presence, severity, and duration of a number of symptoms. Modifications of the K-SADS have been used to assess the entire spectrum of DSM-III-R disorders. In contrast, the DISC is highly structured, can be used by lay interviewers, and was developed primarily for epidemiological studies. If possible, supplemental interviews with at least one parent should be used to confirm diagnosis and obtain additional information that is clinically useful.

Questionnaires

The predominant method for assessing the symptoms and severity of depression has been paper-and-pencil questionnaires. There is a broad range of these instruments that have been developed for use with adolescents. With such measures, cutoff scores are often used to identify "depressed" individuals.

These instruments are frequently used by clinicians because they are easy to administer; some require only brief instructions and a total administration and scoring time of 15-20 minutes. Three of the most widely used instruments for adolescents are the Beck Depression Inventory (BDI; Beck, Ward, Mendelson, Mock, and Erbaugh, 1961), the Reynolds Adolescent Depression Scale (RADS; Reynolds and Coats, 1986), and the Center for Epidemiological Studies; Depression Scale (CES-D; Radloff, 1977). The CES-D is the "Mood Questionnaire" that adolescents fill out at the beginning and end of the course. The BDI and the CES-D were developed using adult populations. Although adaptations for children and adolescents have been developed (e.g., Chiles, Miller, and Cox, 1980; Weissman, Orvaschel, and Padian, 1980, respectively), the adult versions seem to be adequate as long as adolescent norms are used for clinical decision-making. For example, in a number of studies (e.g., Roberts, Andrews, Lewinsohn, and Hops, in press), the mean CES-D score for normal adolescents 14 to 18 years of age was above the accepted cutoff score for clinical depression among adults (the mean score for adolescents was 19 vs. a cutoff score of 16 for adults). Thus, normal adolescents seem to report significantly more depressive symptoms than adults; however, the higher scores do not necessarily mean they are more clinically depressed. The implication is that clinicians must evaluate BDI and CES-D scores subjectively to determine whether a problem exists. Studies currently being conducted at the Oregon Research Institute are validating the BDI and CES-D against DSM-III-R diagnosis based on K-SADS interviews (Roberts, Lewinsohn, and Seeley, 1990).

Problems Associated with Depression

Adolescent depression is associated with a number of personal and environmental difficulties that include engaging in fewer pleasant activities, suicidal ideation, problems with academic achievement, depressogenic cognitions, and increases in stressful events and interpersonal conflicts. It is becoming increasingly clear that these difficulties are risk factors for depression, and therefore should be closely monitored.

Pleasant Activities

Studies have consistently shown that depressed individuals engage in fewer pleasant activities and more unpleasant activities than do nondepressed individuals (Lewinsohn and Graf, 1973). One of the treatment components of the Adolescent Coping with Depression Course involves increasing the adolescent's level of pleasant activities. Several scales are available for assessing pleasant activities: the Adolescent Activities Checklist (Cole, Kelley, and Carey, 1988), and an adaptation of the Pleasant Event Schedule (PES; MacPhillamy and Lewinsohn, 1982) that has been developed for adolescents. The PES is an integral part of the course and is routinely filled out during the intake interview to identify activities for each adolescent to increase. (A copy of the adolescent version of the PES is provided in the *Student Workbook*, and a computerized scoring program is available from the publisher.)

Suicidal Ideation

Clinicians involved in the diagnosis and treatment of depressive behavior need to assess the risk of suicide and take appropriate preventive steps. It has been shown that suicidal ideation occurs more frequently in both females and males with a diagnosis of major depression (Andrews and Lewinsohn, 1989). Furthermore, the absence of suicidal ideation in an otherwise dysphoric adolescent is associated with a decrease in dysphoria one month later (Hops, Lewinsohn, Andrews, and Roberts, in press). Estimates of suicidal ideation can be obtained from the K-SADS interview and from questionnaire data. The K-SADS provides information about the number of discrete gestures or suicide attempts, and ratings of lethality and intent. Several scales have also been developed for rating suicidal ideation and intent. These include the Scale for Suicidal Ideation (Beck, Kovacs, and Weissman, 1979) and the Scale for Suicidal Intent (Beck, Morris, and Beck, 1974), developed for adults but useful for adolescents, and the Suicidal Ideation Questionnaire for adolescents (SIQ; Reynolds, 1987). Any indication of suicidal ideation should be follow up with probes to evaluate its significance.

Academic Achievement

Several studies have demonstrated a relationship between academic achievement and depression (Blechman, McEnroe, Carella, and Audette, 1986; Nolen-Hoeksma, Seligman, and Girgus, 1986). The evidence suggests that poor academic achievement can be either an antecedent or a consequence of depression. It is relatively easy to evaluate academic achievement. If the adolescent is in a school setting, standardized achievement test scores should be available (e.g., Metropolitan Achievement Test). Additional information can be obtained from school records, the adolescent, parents, or school personnel.

Depressogenic Cognitions

The cognitive functions that have been shown to relate to adult depression fall into four general categories: 1) low self-esteem and self-deprecating thoughts; 2) irrational beliefs that cause the individual to overreact emotionally and negative cognitive distortions of experiences; 3) negative attributions, which include the adolescent blaming him- or herself for failures; and 4) reduced rates of self-reinforcement. Several scales have been developed (primarily for adults) to assess these cognitive functions: 1) the Self-Esteem Scale (Rosenberg, 1979), 2) the Dysfunctional Attitude Scale (Weissman and Beck, 1978) and the Subjective Probability Scale (Muñoz and Lewinsohn, 1976), 3) the Children's Attributional Style Questionnaire (Seligman, Peterson, Kaslow, Tanenbaum, Alloy, and Abramson, 1984), and 4) the Self-Reinforcement Attitude Questionnaire (Heiby, 1983). Brief adaptations of these scales have been developed at the Oregon Research Institute for each category except attributional style; norms are available for adolescents 14 to 18 years of age.

Environmental Factors

It has been hypothesized that a number of environmental factors are involved in the development of depressive disorders. For example, depressed people experience a greater number of aversive environmental events than nondepressed individuals and are more sensitive to them (Paykel et al., 1969; Lewinsohn and Talkington, 1979). External stressors can disrupt an individual's adaptive functioning and initiate a chain of events that leads to an increase in depressive symptoms and/or to a depressive episode (Lewinsohn, Hoberman, Teri, and Hautzinger, 1985). A comprehensive assessment of environmental factors should not only focus on the occurrence of key events, but on the way in which the individual perceives those events. Several different instruments have been developed for this purpose.

Macro and micro stressors. External factors associated with increased stress have been conceptualized as macro and micro aversive events. The term "macro stressors" refers to major life events such as the death of a loved one, being transferred to a new school, or failing a grade. The term "micro stressors" refers to the minor daily hassles that tend to have less immediate impact but occur more frequently and can lead to increased levels of stress over time. Two brief scales have been developed at the Oregon Research Institute to assess macro and micro stressors. The macro scale consists of 15 items that sample the events that happened to the adolescent and his or her family and friends during the last year. This scale is an adaptation of two frequently used scales: the Schedule of Recent Experience (Holmes and Rahe, 1967) and the Life Events Schedule (Sandler and Block, 1979). The micro scale consists of 20 items that sample social and nonsocial daily hassles. This scale is an adaptation of the Unpleasant Events Schedule (Lewinsohn, Mermelstein, Alexander, and MacPhillamy, 1984).

Social Conflict. The social-interactional context has been shown to play a significant role in the lives of depressed individuals (Biglan, Hops, and Sherman, 1988; Coyne, Kessler et al., 1987; Youngren and Lewinsohn, 1980). More conflict occurs in families with depressed members than in nondepressed families (Hops et al., 1987). Moreover, chronically dysphoric adolescents perceive more conflict and less cohesiveness in the family and have a more negative view of their parents (Hops, Lewinsohn, Andrews, and Roberts, in press). Thus, it is important to assess the extent of conflict and cohesion in the families of depressed adolescents.

Several measures of family conflict are available. These include the Family Environment Scale (FES; Moos, 1974), which contains scales for both conflict and cohesion. The Issues Checklist (IC; Robin and Weiss, 1980) asks both the adolescent and parent to rate the occurrence, frequency, and intensity of parent-adolescent discussions for 45 different issues. The checklist is most useful if it is filled out by both the adolescent and his or her parents. The checklist is clinically useful because it identifies specific issues that generate conflict within the family, and these topics can then be addressed in therapy. The Issues Checklist has been incorporated into the sessions of the Adolescent Coping with Depression Course that deal with problem solving and negotiation. Two other instruments have been developed at the Oregon Research Institute to provide independent estimates of support/conflict from each parent: the Mother Support Scale and the Father Support Scale.

We recommend that the following instruments be used during the initial intake procedure to determine the significance of the problem and the adolescent's potential for the group procedure. Several instruments could also be administered during intake and again following treatment to determine the outcome. The intake should include a clinical interview using a standardized procedure such as the K-SADS or an informal interview by the therapist to assess the level of depression and to identify specific areas of difficulty. A brief self-report instrument (requiring no more than five or ten minutes to administer) such as the BDI or CES-D should also be used. As mentioned earlier, any indication of suicidal ideation should be followed up with further probes. The PES is routinely filled out by all adolescents who enroll in the course. The schedule should be completed before the first session. The Issues Checklist is another instrument that can be administered during intake to assess the extent of family conflict. Although this checklist is filled out in Session 12 of the course, initial assessment can be compared with post-treatment assessment to evaluate the effect on family relationships.

At the therapist's discretion, the scales noted earlier in this chapter could also be administered during intake to assess depressogenic cognitions, family cohesion, and environmental stress. Norms for many of these scales have been developed at the Oregon Research Institute as part of a large epidemiological study; copies of the instruments and norms can be obtained by writing to: The Oregon Adolescent Depression Project, 1715 Franklin Blvd., Eugene, OR 97403-1983.

Summary

The instruments described in this chapter can be used to assess depressive symptoms and to identify risk factors that may be causally related to depression or that may be maintaining the depressive symptoms. There will be considerable variability within a group of adolescents. Clinicians must therefore evaluate each case independently to determine the severity of the adolescent's depression and the risk of suicide, and to distinguish other factors that may be important for therapy. The assessment battery used for each adolescent does not have to be comprehensive, but the clinician should sample suspected problem areas. Assessments should be routinely conducted before and after treatment to determine whether each adolescent has become less depressed and to evaluate whether there have been corresponding changes in the risk factors for that individual.

Sources for Assessment Instruments

The Beck Depression Inventory (BDI) is available from The Psychological Corporation, 555 Academic Court, San Antonio, TX 78204-2498).

The Reynolds Adolescent Depression Scale (RADS) and the Suicidal Ideation Questionnaire (SIQ) are available from Psychological Assessment Resources, P.O. Box 998, Odessa, FL 33556.

CHAPTER 3
Recruiting Participants

This chapter provides guidelines and suggestions for recruiting participants for the Adolescent Coping with Depression Course. The course is based on a group format designed to accommodate four to eight participants. Since one or two adolescents may drop out of the program, and the course is a time-limited intervention with restricted membership (that is, new participants should not be admitted to the group after it has started), approximately six to ten depressed adolescents must be prepared to enter into a treatment group at the same time. In many settings it may be difficult to find this many depressed adolescents without some active recruitment. Recent research indicates that very few depressed adolescents seek treatment on their own (Lewinsohn, Hops, Roberts, and Seeley, 1988), which suggests that recruitment efforts must be vigorous and should include an active outreach component.

The inclusion and exclusion criteria for course participants are also reviewed in this chapter. The criteria employed in our research investigations, which focused on evaluating the efficacy of this intervention with a relatively "pure" group of depressed adolescents, are presented first. This is followed with a discussion of how these standards can be modified for use in clinical settings.

Referral Sources

Recruiting participants for the course often requires a multifaceted approach that utilizes a variety of referral sources. In this section, three major sources of referrals are examined: school and health professionals, media contacts, and former participants.

School and Health Professionals

The most consistent source of referrals for the course has been high school counselors and school psychologists. Most school districts have an office that coordinates mental health services for students. We have found that the best approach is to contact these offices and arrange to have a meeting with the staff. During the meeting, we describe the Adolescent Coping with Depression Course and our research program. If the staff seems receptive to the idea of encouraging students to enroll in the course, we provide copies of the brochures and posters we have developed for distribution to adolescents and their parents (see Appendix 1). On occasion, we provide consultation to school counselors or psychologists on individual cases, and make assessment recommendations for screening or diagnosing affective disorders. Offering this assistance fosters a good working relationship and gives us an opportunity to help school personnel develop a better understanding of the nature of adolescent depression.

We also recommend sending announcements to community mental agencies and to professionals such as psychologists, psychiatrists, social workers, counselors, and physicians (pediatricians, family practitioners, and specialists in adolescent medicine and/or mental health). While we have had relatively few referrals from professionals as a group, this is probably due to the fact that our research protocol often excludes adolescents who are receiving other forms of treatment from participating in the course. However, these research-based restrictions on enrollment may not be necessary or appropriate when the course is offered in clinical settings such as schools, clinics, and hospitals. In these settings, the course is likely to include adolescents referred by private practitioners who would also provide individual treatment as necessary. On those occasions when our research protocol has allowed adolescents to participate in the course concurrent with other treatments, we have received referrals from mental health professionals.

We have developed a bi-monthly newsletter to keep schools, agencies, and mental health professionals informed about the course and the Adolescent Depression Program. This has proven to be a very effective way to provide essential information and maintain our visibility within the community. Each issue of the newsletter announces the starting date of the next group, describes the referral procedures, and reviews questions posed by health professionals and parents. It is our impression that the regular mailings of the newsletter have had a cumulative effect. Professionals receive numerous service announcements (many of which are misplaced or forgotten), but the bi-monthly appearances of our newsletter seems to create a stronger and more lasting impression.

Former Participants

Former participants can be a significant source of referrals. Class reunions for former group members are an appropriate forum for announcing upcoming courses. Another option would be to modify the newsletter intended for professional audiences and distribute it to former participants; the newsletter would announce upcoming groups and indicate that referrals are welcome. Of course, promotions of this type must be carefully worded to avoid pressuring or obligating former participants to make referrals.

Media Resources

The use of advertisements to recruit mental health patients or participants for research studies has a relatively short history. Until recently, the potential for ethical violations in advertising has kept most professional mental health organizations from using media resources for recruitment or advertising. During the last decade, however, media recruitment has become more widely accepted. We view the use of advertising as being consistent with the community outreach orientation that is generally represented by the Adolescent Coping with Depression Course. This section describes the media approaches we have employed to recruit subjects.

Newspaper advertising has been one of the most successful methods for recruiting new research subjects. This generally produces more inquiries than any other method, except school counselor referrals. While we have no data regarding the effect of placement and frequency of advertisements on overall response, we generally try to place at least half of the advertisements in the local daily newspaper, most often in the weekly television guide (since this section is kept around the house longer than the rest of the paper), and we place some smaller advertisements in local high school monthly newspapers. Again, our impression is that the repeated advertising that appears during the recruitment phases of our research project builds public confidence that our program is a legitimate, enduring resource in the community. We currently use newspaper advertisements as our primary means of publicizing the course, since they are effective and relatively inexpensive.

Another strategy we have used is to enlarge our full-page advertisement and create a flier or handout that is used in schools, community centers, and so on. Larger posters (e.g., 24" x 36") can be strategically placed in high traffic areas such as clinic waiting rooms and school corridors. We also circulate a more comprehensive brochure that lists the symptoms of depression and provides a complete description of the course.

Giving public talks or lectures is another way to make people aware that the course is available. These events are often sponsored by a university or medical facility. We also give presentations to health groups and high school health classes, and we organize "Open House" gatherings that are held during evenings or on weekends at the clinic where the course will be conducted.

Finally, we have had some limited experience with television and radio coverage of our program. Because we are a nonprofit organization, stations have occasionally broadcasted Public Service Announcements (PSAs) that describe our program. We have also experimented with a brief series of paid television advertisements. Somewhat surprisingly, none of these methods have produced a significant increase in inquiries, despite the fact that our television advertisements were professionally produced. If anything, the PSAs were slightly more effective than the paid advertisements.

Ethical Considerations

The ethical issues involved in publicizing the course as a treatment for depression must be seriously considered, especially when nontraditional methods of advertising are employed, such as television and radio commercials. Before advertising the course, potential instructors should carefully review the ethical guidelines that have been established for their profession. Psychologists (and other professionals as well) should refer to the "Ethical Principles of Psychologists" and "Standards for Providers of Psychological Services," published by the American Psychological Association (1981). The APA guidelines are quite clear about what can and cannot be done in advertising. Public statements should *not* contain: 1) a false, fraudulent, misleading, deceptive or unfair statement; 2) a misinterpretation of fact or a statement likely to mislead or deceive; 3) a testimonial from a patient; or 4) a statement intended to (or likely to) create false or unjustified expectations of favorable results.

Group leaders must be willing to assume responsibility for their actions and the consequences that follow. Public statements should be accurate and objectively specify the therapist's qualifications as well as what can be expected from the course. A clear description of the course and its purpose should also be included. Sufficient information should be provided so that potential consumers can make informed judgments and choices. It is not appropriate to make promises regarding treatment outcome as part of a publicity campaign, and all claims regarding the course should be handled with professional integrity. Individuals should be given a realistic appraisal of what they might accomplish by participating in the course; building false hopes can be debilitating to a depressed adolescent.

Inclusion and Exclusion Criteria

This section briefly reviews the inclusion and exclusion criteria that we have used to select subjects for our research studies. While some of these criteria may be too restrictive for clinical settings, others have implications for the functioning of treatment groups. It is therefore recommended that each of the following criteria be carefully considered.

Inclusion Criteria

1. Participants must be suffering from a depressive disorder or mood state. This includes adolescents with a diagnosable DSM-III-R affective disorder (e.g., major depression), as well as individuals with a less severe and perhaps subdiagnostic affective disturbance.

2. Participants must be 14 to 18 years of age (grades 9 through 12 inclusive). We have been asked to provide treatment for adolescents 12 and 13 years of age, or even younger. After a few attempts in the pilot stages of our intervention program, plans to include these younger adolescents in the group treatment were abandoned. One reason for restricting enrollment to older adolescents is that participants must be able to understand and apply the concepts presented in the course. In particular, the constructive thinking and communication sessions often prove to be too difficult for younger adolescents. Another reason for restricting enrollment is that group cohesion is an important part of the group therapy process, and this is compromised if the age range is too broad. The emotional and intellectual differences within the age range allowed by our criteria can sometimes be quite significant, and including younger adolescents would only exacerbate this potential problem.

Nonetheless, it may be very worthwhile to offer a version of the Adolescent Coping with Depression Course to a homogenous group of younger adolescents (e.g., just 12- and 13-year-olds). This would undoubtedly require some modification of the content and pace of the course. For example, the terminology and concepts would have to be simplified, the pace of the sessions would have to be slowed down, and so on.

We have also been asked to provide treatment for adolescents who are older than 18. This may be due to the fact that adult treatment resources are more readily available for these older adolescents and/or because we clearly state that the treatment program is exclusively designed for adolescents 14 to 18 years of age. We have not attempted to include these older adolescents in our treatment groups.

3. Participants must be able to read at or above a 7th grade level. Adolescents are given a lengthy workbook that is integrated with the course exercises and homework assignments. Poor reading skills would interfere with mastering the material presented in the course and might have the iatrogenic effect of setting up the reading-impaired adolescent for another failure experience. We strongly recommend screening all potential participants for adequate reading skills before enrolling them in the course. Instructors may need to provide individual assistance to adolescents whose reading level is significantly below the criteria we have established.

Exclusion Criteria

1. One or more current DSM-III-R diagnoses of bipolar disorder with mania, bipolar disorder with hypomania, panic disorder, drug or alcohol abuse/dependence, conduct disorder, or a current or past history of schizophrenia and/or schizo-affective disorder. These criteria are considered to be the most restrictive from a clinical perspective, especially in view of the research that indicates high co-morbidity of these and other mental disorders with adolescent and adult depression (e.g., Lehmann, 1985; Maser and Clonniger, 1989; Lewinsohn, Hops, Roberts, and Seeley, 1988). Nonetheless, each of the disorders listed above should be carefully considered when reviewing potential participants. Depressed adolescents with these co-morbid disorders may require additional forms of treatment in conjunction with participating in the course (e.g., lithium carbonate for bipolar adolescents and substance abuse programs for teenagers with drug and alcohol problems). Another factor is that the behaviors exhibited by these adolescents can be disruptive to the group, sometimes to the point of jeopardizing the therapeutic process. In these cases, it would be better to screen out disruptive teenagers before the group begins.

2. The presence of organic brain syndrome or mental retardation. Again, these criteria are necessary to ensure that the adolescent will be able to master the skills presented in the course.

3. Symptoms requiring immediate treatment and/or hospitalization, or extreme risk of suicide. Group therapy by itself is not a recommended treatment modality for adolescents experiencing acute psychiatric turmoil. These adolescents would be better served by individual therapy and/or placement in a more intensive environment (e.g., residential care, day treatment, or hospitalization), where their crisis status can be regularly assessed as treatment is administered. The Adolescent Coping with Depression Course, in contrast, does not provide for routine assessment of crisis-related problems, and teenagers are often reluctant to discuss suicidal or psychotic thoughts and behaviors that are unusual in a group setting, regardless of how cohesive the group may be.

Recommended Sequence of Recruitment

Finally, good timing and adequate planning are necessary to ensure that the Adolescent Coping with Depression Course runs smoothly. We have found that a tremendous amount of effort and coordination is necessary to set up a successful course. A recommended timeline for recruiting and screening participants is briefly summarized below.

If this is the first time the course is being offered at a clinic or school, it will take a minimum of four months to generate interest in the program within the community. During the first two months (three and four months before the starting date), contact professional groups, give talks and lectures, meet with school personnel, and begin mailing a newsletter. Then, in the remaining two months before the group starts, continue to generate community interest and begin to recruit participants directly through the use of newspaper advertisements and radio and television PSAs.

Intake interviews should be conducted no more than three to four weeks before the course starts. The first stage of the intake interview involves screening adolescents to make sure they fit the criteria for participating in the course. It is up to the therapist to determine which assessment methods will be used for this screening (Chapter 2 provides a detailed description of the instruments currently available). The recommended procedure is to use a combination of a diagnostic interview and a self-report questionnaire such as the Beck Depression Inventory (Beck et al., 1961). Adolescents who meet the criteria for inclusion in the course should be given a *Student Workbook* and asked to fill out the PES contained in the appendix before they come to the first session. It is also important to answer any questions the adolescents may have about the course, and to reassure them that they will have a positive experience.

CHAPTER 4
General Issues in Conducting Groups

Even a cursory glance through the course material in this manual reveals highly structured sessions that involve lectures, discussions, activities, and homework assignments. Although the directives to group leaders are very specific and many of the problems encountered in running groups are addressed within the course sessions, there are some general issues that are not covered. This chapter discusses these issues and associated problems, and offers solutions where appropriate.

Group Cohesiveness

In the present context, the term *group cohesiveness* refers to the common bond between its members, and the shared sense of commitment and belonging that develops as participants spend time together. It is an index of the extent to which participants enjoy being in the group and feel that the other members care about them, understand them, and are their friends. It should not be surprising that group cohesiveness is an important factor in achieving a successful outcome for adolescents enrolled in the course. It plays a significant role not only in mediating the obvious behavioral benefits associated with involvement in a group (e.g., it offers a variety of resources for role playing, feedback, modeling, and social interaction), but also in terms of intangibles such as empathy for shared experiences and identification with one another as individuals attempting to recover from depression. It has been shown that group cohesiveness is one of the best predictors of outcome for adults who have participated in the Coping with Depression Course (Hoberman, Lewinsohn, and Tilson, 1988).

There are several ways to foster group cohesiveness. The 10-minute social break that is routinely scheduled halfway through each session is one of the most straightforward, yet effective methods. These breaks are particularly important because most of the adolescents do not know one another, and they are usually embarrassed about being in the course; many of them are quiet and shy, and at the beginning of the first session there are often very few spontaneous interactions. However, some tentative but significant socializing is usually initiated during the first break. These interactions can be enhanced by making snacks available (food is a "social facilitator") and by asking the adolescents to practice using specific social skills with one another during the break.

Another method for increasing group cohesiveness involves pairing up adolescents who seem compatible (same age, similar interests, etc.) for the

31

early role-playing exercises. These "compatible pairs" are kept together for several sessions to help warm up the group, then leaders are encouraged to rotate team partners throughout the rest of the course to ensure that the adolescents have some contact with the other members of the group. This minimizes the problem of exclusive cliques forming within the group, which could lead to conflict or antagonism.

Leaders should track group cohesiveness over the duration of the treatment program to ensure that it continues to develop as the course progresses. A relatively brief self-report questionnaire is used in our research project to measure group cohesiveness; this is a modified version of the Yalom Group Cohesiveness Questionnaire (Yalom, 1970), which consists of 11 items such as "If you could replace members of your group with other 'ideal group members,' how many would you trade?" The recommended procedure is for therapists to assess cohesiveness at the end of Sessions 3, 8, and 16. If assessment reveals that group cohesiveness is low, leaders should try to improve the situation by using some procedures such as those outlined above.

Trust and Rapport

Another important component of a successful outcome is developing trust and rapport between the leader and the adolescents, and between the teenagers themselves. Several aspects of the course are designed to enhance trust. In the first session, adolescents are told that the information shared by group members is confidential (this is one of the "ground rules" for the course). While there are some exceptions to the confidentiality rule for group leaders (e.g., medical emergencies and situations in which teenagers are judged to be dangerous to themselves or to someone else), adolescents are encouraged to regard the sessions as a safe place to talk about their problems and concerns.

It is also important for adolescents to have the option of withholding private information. During recruitment and intake interviews, teenagers often express the concern that they will be forced to "bare their souls" in the group sessions. Letting the adolescents know that they can decide whether they want to reveal personal information makes them more likely to participate in a group, and ultimately much more comfortable when they do decide to disclose something personal.

Building rapport between the therapist and the adolescents is a little more complicated. Some therapists may try to become "one of the gang" by dressing and talking like a teenager. In general, we discourage this approach to building rapport, because it blurs the important therapeutic distinction between patient and therapist, and it degrades the leader's authority which may be critical if the teenagers become disruptive. The final and most persuasive

32

argument against this approach is the reaction of the adolescents, who most often view such attempts by adults with disdain.

In general, we suggest that therapists use a friendly, understanding, but firm approach with adolescent participants. Leaders should try to have fun with the activities and at the same time maintain control of the group and the amount of time spent on tasks. It is also important to be relatively nonjudgmental about the way the adolescents dress and behave, unless there is evidence that a negative behavior (or lack of prosocial behavior) is involved in maintaining their depression.

We have found that adolescents respond very well to being treated like adults. Therapists are encouraged to ask adolescents for their opinions, to value their suggestions, and to let them set their own limits on sharing personal information. By treating them with the same respect as we would adult group participants, we obtain cooperation and develop rapport in the majority of cases.

Homework Problems

The homework assignments can be a potential source of difficulty for many participants. A large percentage of the depressed adolescents who have enrolled in the course report ongoing difficulty completing their regular school assignments. The prospect of having semiweekly homework assignments in the course only compounds the problem.

Our approach to reducing anxiety about the homework assignments is to emphasize that: 1) the homework is for them, not for us (it helps them gain control over their depressed moods); 2) in contrast to school homework, the assignments are often related to real-life situations that are bothering them (e.g., conflict with parents, social isolation, tension or fears); 3) the course assignments are usually brief and are easy to integrate into their daily routines; and 4) the homework is completely voluntary, although the leader reviews everyone's assignments at the beginning of every session. Making the homework assignments voluntary reflects our commitment to treating the adolescents as responsible young adults. It is also an acknowledgement of the fact that we cannot *force* them to do the homework. Nonetheless, participants are asked about their homework at each session, including those who have not completed any of their earlier assignments. Sometimes our persistence is rewarded as the adolescents realize we are not going to drop the subject.

To further promote homework completion, especially for those adolescents who chronically fail to complete (or even begin) their assignments, we routinely encourage them to work on the uncompleted portion of their assignment during the early part of each session when homework is reviewed.

If necessary, the forms for tracking behaviors or thoughts are completed retrospectively, at least for the past few days. In this manner, we never acquiesce to passive withdrawal from the activities of the group, but continue to gently push adolescents toward active involvement.

Attendance

Attendance rates for adolescent groups in our first treatment outcome study (Lewinsohn, Clarke, Hops, and Andrews, 1990) averaged 89% across all subjects who completed the course; this means participants attended an average of 12.5 out of the 14 sessions contained in the earlier version of the course. These attendance rates seem adequate in the sense that they are associated with significant improvement in course participants, but we never have been fully satisfied with them. We have tried a variety of techniques to increase attendance, but have had little success. The following is a description of the procedures that are implemented when an adolescent does not show up for a session.

First, the group leader calls each absent adolescent either on the evening of the missed session or the day after. The leader expresses concern that the teenager did not come to the group, asks how he or she is doing, and inquires about the reason(s) for not showing up. The leader emphasizes how much the teenager was missed by the rest of the group and asks when he or she will be returning. If several sessions are missed, then the leader also calls the adolescent's parent(s) to ask for their assistance in making sure that the teenager attends regularly.

Second, the leader arranges to have an individual meeting with each absent adolescent, either just before or just after the next session, to cover the main points of the missed session(s). This minimizes the effect that falling behind on the material might have on future attendance.

We have found that the attendance of the adolescents appears to be more consistent when their parents are enrolled in the companion course for parents. This is true even in our treatment outcome studies in which some parents are randomly assigned to a parent group and others are not (the parents do not have a choice regarding enrollment, although obviously they do choose whether or not to attend). We are not certain why parent participation improves the attendance of the adolescents. Because of random assignment, any bias in selection can be ruled out (e.g., that the more involved parents will both enroll in the parent group and be more regular in bringing their adolescents to their group). Another possible explanation is that the parents develop an emotional and intellectual commitment to the treatment approach, or that the parents acquire a better understanding of their adolescent's problems by participating in a parent group. A more mundane explanation is that when both adolescents and parents are attending groups with a common destination on the same day, there are fewer conflicts regarding transportation arrangements.

While this entire section has been devoted to outlining ways to improve attendance, it is instructive to examine the underlying (and often unchallenged) assumption that increased attendance actually does contribute to a successful outcome. That is, do adolescents who attend more regularly recover from depression more often? In an exploratory series of regression analyses (Clarke, Lewinsohn, Hops, and Andrews, 1989) designed to identify variables which predict greater pre- to post-treatment improvement among adolescents in our first treatment outcome study (Lewinsohn, Clarke, Hops, Andrews, and Williams, 1990), we found that adolescent attendance *did not* significantly predict recovery from depression. Although this data is preliminary, the findings fail to explicitly support the expected link between attendance and improvement. However, because these results are based on a relatively small sample of 40 adolescents, they should be regarded with some skepticism until we have had an opportunity to cross-validate them on a much larger treatment outcome sample. A study is currently in progress with a projected total of 200 adolescents (Lewinsohn, Clarke, and Hops, 1990). If the same results are obtained, the following questions become relevant: Is there a minimum number of sessions which are necessary to obtain a significant therapeutic benefit from the course? If attendance does not make an important contribution to successful outcome, then what is the mechanism through which therapeutic change occurs? These questions, and others like them, address some of the basic underlying issues of psychotherapy.

Drop Outs

Much to our surprise, we have had very little trouble with subjects dropping out of the course. Once adolescents have made the commitment to attend the first few sessions, we have had reasonable success in retaining them. In our second treatment outcome study (Lewinsohn, Clarke, Hops, Andrews, and Williams, 1990) we had a drop-out rate of only 12%, despite some very reluctant adolescents who were initially compelled to attend by their parents.

For reluctant or resistant adolescents, we use the following approach. First, we acknowledge their concerns and agree that they will be the final judge as to whether the course is appropriate for them. At the same time, because they really don't know what the course is all about, we make the following proposal: we ask them to agree to attend a minimum of three sessions so they can find out what the group is like. If they want to withdraw from the group at the end of this trial period, the leader will help the adolescent and his or her parents locate other treatment resources. This strategy seems to work well with most adolescents because it reduces their anxiety about losing control. To date, no one has withdrawn from the course at the end of the trial period, although a few of these resistant adolescents have simply stopped attending the sessions. Overall, however, this approach has clearly persuaded many adolescents to participate in the course who otherwise would not have enrolled.

When the parents are involved in the program, we have noticed that a small proportion of the families begin to "fade away" as the group progresses; their attendance becomes more sporadic until they no longer show up. For these families, the initial investment in treatment does not seem strong enough to carry them through to the end. While this may simply be a mismatch between our approach and the needs of the family, it is our impression that many of these families are crisis reactive; that is, they seek immediate assistance when a crisis surfaces, but lose the motivation to remain in treatment once the perceived crisis has passed. Even though the adolescent may still be depressed and at risk for other difficulties, the post-crisis clinical picture is one that the family may find familiar: a quiet, withdrawn adolescent, who lacks self-motivation. We believe that the key to keeping these families involved is to call them periodically and gently remind them that the adolescent is very likely to have recurring problems with depression unless the family completes the course or receives some other from of treatment.

Following the Protocol

If the spectrum of possible interventions ranges from very spontaneous and unstructured at one pole to very structured at the other pole, the Adolescent Coping with Depression Course would be placed near the latter pole. While the highly organized format makes it easy for therapists to conduct the course, there is very little allowance for unstructured time during the sessions. Some adolescents and/or leaders may wish there were more opportunities to discuss topics at greater length or to spend additional time on selected skills and activities (or even to digress into other skill areas and personal issues). A question we are often asked is "How closely must I follow the protocol for your intervention?"

For research purposes, we have been very consistent about following the content and pace of the sessions as they are presented in this manual, and the outcome studies summarized in Chapter 7 reflect this approach to treatment. In clinical settings, however, it may not be necessary to follow the protocol as rigidly. It is up to the therapist's discretion to change the pace and content of the sessions to meet the needs of the group (or the individual). Some therapists may want to include additional role plays or discuss related topics that are not covered in the manual. Other therapists may decide to use selected portions of the treatment program or offer shorter sessions by stopping at the break. It is difficult, however, to predict what impact these and other possible modifications of the course might have on therapeutic outcome. This topic is discussed in more detail in the next chapter.

CHAPTER 5
Variations in the Use of the Course

Although the Adolescent Coping with Depression Course is designed for use with groups of four to eight adolescents, other variations are possible depending upon the situation and related goals. With some modification, the course could be used on an individual basis with depressed adolescents and/or in conjunction with other types of treatment (e.g., individual psychotherapy, medications, etc.), with special populations such as adolescents with serious reading problems, or with nondepressed teenagers as a preventive program.

Use on an Individual Basis

There are many settings in which it would be difficult to assemble a group of depressed adolescents at any one time. For example, clinicians working in private practice or small clinic settings typically see a wide variety of patients, and this particular treatment program may be appropriate for only a few of them. In this case, the course could be modified so that it could be offered on an individual basis.

The most significant changes would involve the role-playing exercises designed for pairs of adolescents. For these exercises, the leader would have to assume a dual role as therapist and role-playing partner. During the communication skills exercises this would mean playing the part of the other teenager, and in the family problem-solving sessions it would mean taking the role of the adolescent's parents. It is possible to do this successfully, but it would require some additional preparation on the part of the therapist.

One of the most salient advantages to offering the course on an individual basis is that it can be customized to address the specific needs of each adolescent. For example, if increasing pleasant events is particularly important, more time could be spent on that skill area. In a similar vein, if the adolescent has good communication skills, a brief assessment of those skills may be all that is necessary before moving on to the next lesson.

Using Selected Modules

Since the course offers curriculum-based instruction, modules can be selected to address the skill deficits of an individual client (as mentioned above) or a group of clients with similar needs. For example, if family conflict is a problem for several adolescents and their parents, the therapist could form a treatment group and administer the sessions that deal with communication, problem-solving, and negotiation. Similarly, the modules that offer instruction on controlling negative and irrational thoughts could be used with a group of teenagers with depressogenic thinking styles. Regardless of which modules are selected, Session 1 should be retained since it provides an overview of the ground rules for the entire course.

Modifications for Specific Settings and Special Populations

Many of the skills taught in the course are essential for general adaptive functioning. Consequently, there are a number of ways in which the course could be used with adolescents who may not be suffering from clinical depression. For example, the course could be offered as a "life skills" class for normal teenagers or as a preventive program for teenagers who are at risk for depression. With some modification, the skills could also be taught to special populations with sensory or developmental handicaps. The following is a discussion of some of the possibilities.

High school health classes. In most high schools, students are required to attend health classes. The trend seems to be that an increasingly wide range of issues are being addressed in these classes. Consequently, health classes are a promising vehicle for teaching both high-risk and normal adolescents to recognize the danger signals of depression and for helping them to develop related coping skills. Specific aspects of the Adolescent Coping with Depression Course could be used to develop the curriculum for a mini-series on depression. Depending on the number of class periods available, the content might consist of two to four lectures on the symptoms of depression, how students can recognize the symptoms in themselves and their peers, and common causes and risk factors. A videotape with accompanying materials is currently being produced for this purpose. (Institutions and individuals who have purchased this manual will be contacted by the publisher when it becomes available.)

Psychiatric hospitals (inpatient and aftercare). The course is appropriate for use in psychiatric hospitals or other group residential facilities for adolescents. Some changes would be necessary since there are limitations on the activities allowed in such settings. For example, the acceptable range of pleasant activities would have to be approved by the staff, and relevant hospital situations and activities might have to be incorporated into the role-playing exercises. Staff members could also be involved in helping the adolescents practice their communication, problem-solving, and negotiation skills. Certainly, the skills taught in the course would continue to be useful to the adolescents after they have been discharged from the hospital.

Special populations. Some modules of the course could be employed, under controlled conditions, with adolescents who are developmentally delayed or learning disabled. For example, it would be difficult for adolescents with serious reading problems to complete many of the assignments and activities in the workbook, but the group leaders (or assistants) could read the workbook material out loud and have the adolescents respond orally if necessary. The course could also be modified for developmentally delayed students. However, the material would have to be substantially simplified and some of the more complex tasks would have to be omitted. Oral presentations may also be necessary depending upon the reading level of the students.

With some relatively straightforward modifications in teaching methods, the course could be offered to adolescents who are deaf or blind. Questions and specific tasks would be administered and answered orally for blind students. Deaf students could do all of the written work as described, but would need a group leader who could use sign language or other appropriate methods of communication.

Booster Sessions

It is becoming increasingly clear that it may be necessary to have some ongoing contact with course participants to prevent the recurrence of depressive symptoms. Long-term studies indicate that the relapse rate among adults is particularly high during the first year after treatment. We are currently investigating several different follow-up procedures that can be employed to help adolescents maintain treatment gains.

The basic approach involves conducting one or more booster sessions to briefly review the skills taught in the course and monitor each adolescent's progress. The sessions can be offered on an individual basis or to groups of adolescents. During the sessions, participants are asked to describe their current situations, and specific problems are addressed by emphasizing the relevant skills and doing some role plays to illustrate how to apply them. Positive changes should receive attention during the booster sessions as well, and getting together as a group makes it possible for the adolescents to renew their connections with one another, which can be a valuable resource for ongoing support.

Another variation of the booster session model is to contact adolescents by telephone or through the mail. Because the procedures are relatively familiar and the adolescents can refer to their workbooks, the leader may be able to offer assistance without extensive involvement and hands-on instruction.

Summary

The skills taught in the Adolescent Coping with Depression Course have the potential for a wide range of applications. Although the modifications discussed in this chapter have not been empirically tested, it seems reasonable to assume that the course would have some utility for a variety of adolescents in diverse settings. We are looking forward to receiving feedback from clinicians regarding their successes and failures in using variations of the course.

CHAPTER 6
Theoretical Background

This chapter provides a succinct overview of the theoretical underpinnings of the Adolescent Coping with Depression Course. Since the course is a "cognitive-behavioral" intervention, the chapter begins with a general definition of the term. This is followed with a review of the studies that have investigated the efficacy of cognitive-behavioral interventions with adults. The relationship between theory and treatment is examined next, and the implications for the theoretical foundations of the course are discussed. The final section of the chapter provides a brief history of the development of the Adolescent Coping with Depression Course.

Cognitive-Behavioral Interventions

The term *cognitive-behavioral intervention* encompasses a number of conceptually and methodologically diverse treatment approaches. It includes treatments based on cognitive theories of depression (Rush, Beck, Kovacs, and Hollon, 1977), self-control theories of depression (Rehm, 1977), behavioral formulations (Lewinsohn, Youngren, and Grosscup, 1979; McLean, Ogsdon, and Grauer, 1973; McLean and Hakstian, 1979), interpersonal interaction theories of depression (Weissman, Prusoff, DiMascio, Neu, Goklaney, and Klerman, 1979) and social skills approaches (Bellack, Hersen, and Himmelhoch, 1981; Sanchez, Lewinsohn, and Larson, 1980). While there are many significant differences between each of these treatment approaches, they all assume that the depressed patient has *acquired* maladaptive reaction patterns that can be *unlearned*. Symptoms are viewed as important in their own right rather than considering them to be manifestations of underlying conflicts, and treatments focus on modifying relatively specific behaviors and cognitions rather than on a general reorganization of the patient's personality. All cognitive-behavioral treatments are structured and time limited.

Treatment Efficacy

Studies conducted during the last decade have demonstrated the effectiveness of cognitive-behavioral interventions for the treatment of unipolar depression (DeRubeis and Hollon, 1981; Hoberman and Lewinsohn, 1985; Hollon and Beck, 1987; Lewinsohn, Hoberman, and Clarke, 1989; McLean and Carr, 1989; Sacco and Back, 1985). Investigators have shown that treatment packages involving a variety of cognitive and behavioral tactics are superior to control conditions. Moreover, a number of studies (Beck, Hollon, Young, Bedrosian, and Budenz, 1985; McLean and Hakstian, 1979; Murphy, Simons, Wetzel, and Lustman, 1984) as well as the multi-site NIMH collaborative research program for the treatment of depression (Elkin, Parloff, Hadley, and Autry, 1985) indicate that cognitive-behavioral interventions are at least as effective as antidepressive medication. A meta-analysis of 56 outcome studies of pharmacological and psychotherapeutic treatments of unipolar depression in adults suggested that psychotherapy (most of which was cognitive-behavioral) has an average effectiveness almost twice that of medications (Steinbrueck, Maxwell, and Howard, 1983).

Although there are important differences in methods, the various cognitive-behavioral treatments appear to produce similar outcome results. This uniformity of successful treatment outcomes among these diverse interventions poses an interesting theoretical question. Since all of the treatments were theoretically derived (i.e., they were designed to target the specific cognitions and/or behaviors postulated by a particular theory to be critical antecedents for depression), how could they *all* be effective? Furthermore, while each of these treatments was effective in ameliorating depression, they were not specific in impacting only the intervening target behaviors and/or cognitions at which they were directed. A study by Zeiss, Lewinsohn, and Muñoz (1979) compared the following three treatments: cognitive therapy, pleasant activities (behavioral), and social skills training. The results indicated that while all three treatments were equally effective in reducing the level of depression, the changes in the intervening dependent measures were not treatment specific. In other words, the cognitions of the patients in the social skills treatment changed as much as the cognitions of the patients in the cognitive therapy group, and their social skills were equally changed; the pleasant activities of patients in the behavioral treatment changed as much as the pleasant activities of those in cognitive therapy, and so on.

Critical Components

These results prompted Zeiss and colleagues to advance the following hypotheses about the critical components for a successful short-term, cognitive-behavioral therapy for depression:

1. Therapy should begin with an elaborated, well-planned rationale. This rationale should provide the initial structure that guides the patient to the belief that s/he can control his/her own behavior, and thereby change his/her depression.

2. Therapy should provide training in skills which the patient can use to feel more effective in handling his/her daily life. The skills must be of some significance to the patient and must fit with the rationale that has been presented.

3. Therapy should emphasize the independent use of these skills by the patient outside of the therapy context and must provide enough structure so that the attainment of independent skills is possible for the patient.

4. Therapy should encourage the patient's attribution that improvement in mood was caused by the patient's own increased skillfulness, not by the therapist's skillfulness (Zeiss et al., 1979, pp. 437-438).

The Coping with Depression Course was designed to incorporate these components. The development of the course will be discussed after a brief review of the theoretical structure on which it is based.

Clinical Implications of Depression Theory

From a clinical perspective, the primary purpose of a theory of depression is to provide a conceptual basis for treatment. In specifying the functional relationships between certain antecedent events and the occurrence of depression, a theory represents a statement about the likely reasons for an individual's depression. The theory thus dictates the goals for therapy which, if accomplished, should lead to a reduction in the level of depression.

Initially, the theories developed by Lewinsohn and colleagues focused on the relationship between depression and reinforcement (Lewinsohn, Youngren, and Grosscup, 1979). It was thought that a decrease in positive interactions with the environment (e.g., response-contingent reinforcement) was associated with dysphoria and a reduced rate of behavior (e.g., depression). It was hypothesized that these changes in positive interactions with the environment were due to a lack of, or a reduction in, positive reinforcement or an increase in aversive experiences. Thus, relatively low rates of response-contingent positive reinforcement (positive social interactions, pleasant activities and events, etc.) constituted a critical antecedent for the occurrence of unipolar depression. This led to the prediction that when individuals engage in more positive interactions with their environment their mood will improve, and as they are reinforced by their improved mood they will be more likely to engage in those positive behaviors in the future.

The implication for treatment derived from this initial behavioral model was that depressed individuals should increase the quantity and quality of their positive activities *and* decrease their levels of negative or punishing activities. This approach was used and described in a series of early investigations (Lewinsohn, Weinstein, and Shaw, 1969; Lewinsohn and Shaw, 1969; Lewinsohn and Atwood, 1969; Lewinsohn and Shaffer; 1971; Robinson and Lewinsohn, 1973).

The Integrative Model

Recently, Lewinsohn, Hoberman, Teri, and Hautzinger (1985) have provided a more comprehensive theoretical model of the etiology and maintenance of depression. The model presented in Figure 1 attempts to integrate the findings of recent epidemiological studies (Lewinsohn, Clarke, Hops, Andrews, and Osteen, 1987) and treatment outcome studies (Zeiss et al., 1979) with the phenomenon of self-awareness that has been advanced by social psychologists (Carver and Scheier, 1982).

Figure 1: An Integrative Model of Depression

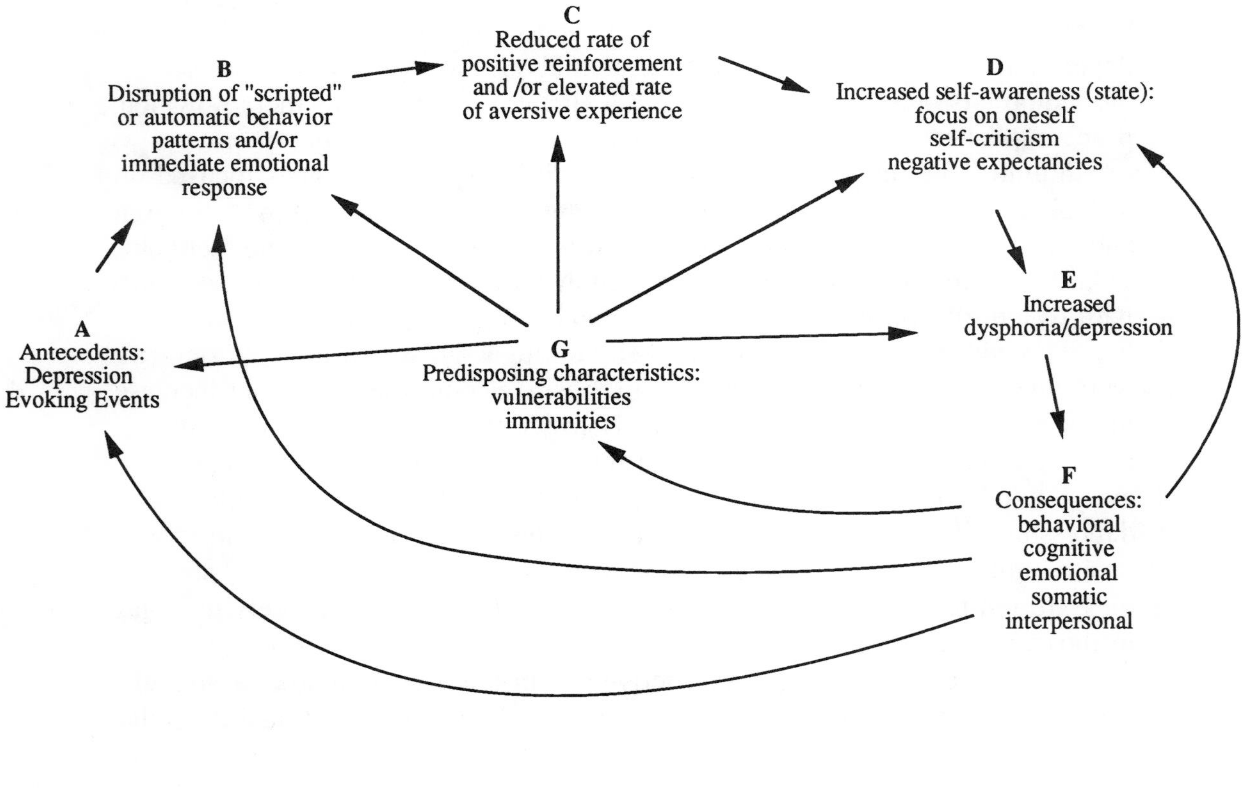

This integrative model suggests that the depressogenic process begins with the occurrence of antecedents or "depression-evoking events." Such stressors initiate the path to a depressive episode to the extent that they disrupt significant positive behavior patterns of individuals. The disruption of these person-environment interaction patterns produces a shift in the quality of the individual's interactions and results in negative emotional response (e.g., dysphoria). As a result, the balance between positive and negative interactions with the environment moves even farther in a negative direction.

A continuing inability to reverse the change in reinforcement is hypothesized to lead to a heightened state of self-awareness. Such a state has been demonstrated to have many negative consequences such as an increase in self-criticism, self-attribution of negative outcomes, intensification of negative affect, and behavioral withdrawal. When this state of self-awareness is elicited, it breaks through the individual's self-protective, self-enhancing cognitive schema (Alloy and Abramson, 1979; Lewinsohn, Mischel, Chaplin, and Barton, 1980) and heightens the individual's awareness of failing to live up to the expected standards for coping. This, in turn, produces a state of further self-denigration and behavioral withdrawal. Finally, the increasing dysphoria is assumed to lead to the behavioral, cognitive, emotional, and interpersonal changes that have previously been shown to be associated with depression. These changes are presumed to "lock" the heightened state of self-awareness and dysphoria into a vicious cycle, which serves to maintain the depressive state.

As a guide for treatment, the integrative model has numerous implications (Lewinsohn, Hoberman, Teri, and Hautzinger [1985] provides a more detailed description of the model). First, it suggests that there are a large number of individual and environmental factors that have an impact on depression. At the same time, it supports the concept that depression can be reduced by changing the person's actions, feelings, thoughts, or environment. While a number of different factors can "cause" depression, none of them may be sufficient or necessary by themselves. The eclectic nature of the Coping with Depression Course (both the adolescent and adult versions) is consistent with this multifactorial position.

Development of the Course

The Adolescent Coping with Depression Course is a descendant of the behavioral treatment approach developed by Lewinsohn and colleagues (1969). The first trial of the group behavioral approach to the treatment of depression was described by Lewinsohn, Weinstein and Alper (1970). The authors created a behaviorally oriented group therapy in which data were collected on specific aspects of the participants' social behavior and its consequences in group interactions during the treatment sessions. Feedback was provided to group members during the individual therapy sessions that were held between sessions. The group meetings were organized as "self-study" groups in which members would be able to learn about their behavior and its consequences on others. During the individual therapy sessions, each member received verbal accounts of his/her own behavior in the group (supported by graphs and data) that identified specific behavioral problems and goals for change. The experience with this initial therapy group study suggested that teaching depressed patients to modify their social behavior might significantly improve their depressed mood. These early therapeutic endeavors also provided support for the behavioral theory of depression.

Two additional aspects of the theoretical foundation of the course should be mentioned. The first aspect is the social learning theory analysis of depression on which the course is based. According to social learning theory (Bandura, 1977), emotional disorders previously considered to be external manifestations of internal (psychic) conflicts, are considered instead to be behaviors that are influenced by the same laws of learning and development that hold for normal behavior. Abnormal behaviors are thus considered to be learned phenomena that influence, and are influenced by, a person's interactions with the environment. A second aspect of our theoretical foundation specifically addresses actions, feelings, and thoughts that have been shown to be functionally related to depression. These include reduced pleasant activities, social-interactional difficulties, problematic cognitions related to depression, and anxiety. Recognizing the multiplicity and heterogeneity of problems experienced by depressed individuals, we have attempted to provide a "smorgasbord" of relevant skills training in the course.

Description of the Adult Course

The adult Coping with Depression Course consists of twelve 2-hour sessions conducted over eight weeks. Sessions are held twice a week for the first four weeks, and once a week for the remaining four weeks. Groups typically consist of six to ten adults (at least 18 years of age) with a single group leader, although two therapists may be used. Follow-up sessions, called "class reunions," are held one month and six months after the course is terminated to help maintain treatment gains and to collect information on improvement or relapse. Like the adolescent version, the adult course focuses on increasing pleasant events, learning relaxation, changing irrational/negative thoughts, practicing social skills, and preventing relapses.

All sessions are highly structured, and an instructor's manual provides scripts, exercises, and guidelines for running the course (Lewinsohn, Antonuccio, Steinmetz-Breckenridge, and Teri, 1984). Each session includes lectures, a review of the homework assignment, discussions, role-play exercises, and structured tasks. A 10-minute break in the middle of each session gives participants opportunities to socialize and to practice the new skills they have learned. In conjunction with the lectures, participants read selected chapters in the book *Control Your Depression* (Lewinsohn, Muñoz, Youngren, and Zeiss, 1986), and fill out the self-monitoring forms in the *Participant Workbook* (Brown and Lewinsohn, 1984a).

CHAPTER 7
Research Findings

This chapter reviews the studies that have evaluated the efficacy of the Coping with Depression Course as a treatment for adults and adolescents.

Efficacy of the Course with Adults

Four outcome studies have been completed to date on the adult Coping with Depression Course (Brown and Lewinsohn, 1984b; Hoberman, Lewinsohn, and Tilson, 1988; Steinmetz, Lewinsohn, and Antonuccio, 1983; Teri and Lewinsohn, 1985). The results of these studies are summarized in Table 1.

Table 1

**Mean Beck Depression Inventory Scores from
Four Treatment Outcome Studies**

Study and Condition	N	Pre-Tx	Post-Tx	Follow Up 1-Month	6-Month
Hoberman, Lewinsohn, & Tilson (1988)					
Class	40	24.4	6.0	7.3	8.5
Brown & Lewinsohn (1984b)					
Class	31	19.8	7.6	6.6	6.4
Individual	15	24.4	9.5	11.1	7.4
Phone	12	20.1	10.8	10.1	9.5
Delayed Control	13	20.5	13.9	—	—
Steinmetz, Lewinsohn, & Antonuccio (1983)					
Class	93	21.1	6.8	6.5	7.9
Teri & Lewinsohn (1985)					
Class	55	19.9	4.7	5.8	5.3
Individual	29	18.2	2.8	5.1	8.0

Depression was assessed through the use of a self-report measure, the Beck Depression Inventory (BDI; Beck, Ward, Mendelson, Mock, and Erbaugh, 1961), and a 2-hour, semi-structured pre-treatment interview, the Schedule for Affective Disorders and Schizophrenia (SADS; Endicott and Spitzer, 1978). A second, shorter version of the interview, the Schedule for Affective Disorders and Schizophrenia, Change Version (SADS-C; Spitzer and Endicott, 1978), was used to measure change from pre-treatment to post-treatment and at follow up.

Brown and Lewinsohn (1984b) compared the Coping with Depression Course to three other conditions: 1) a waiting-list control group, 2) individual tutoring based on the Coping with Depression Course, and 3) a minimal phone contact procedure. As indicated in Table 1, participants in all three active treatment conditions showed substantial improvement. The improvement evident in depressed adults participating in the Coping with Depression Course was substantial at post-treatment, and these gains were maintained at 1-month and 6-month follow-up. The results indicate that there was little difference in efficacy between group and individual treatment. In two other studies (Steinmetz, Lewinsohn, and Antonuccio, 1983; Hoberman et al., 1988), there were significant decreases in pre-treatment and post-treatment BDI scores and lower rates of depression were also noted.

While the results across studies show that a majority of depressed adults are improved at the end of treatment, a significant proportion (approximately 20%) are still depressed at the end of treatment. Still, it would appear that the Coping with Depression Course in its current format is a viable and cost-effective treatment for depressed outpatients. In addition, a pilot study has shown that the course is an effective intervention for depressed inpatients who had been refractory to pharmacological treatment (Antonuccio, Akins, Chatham, Monagin, Tearnan, and Ziegler, 1983).

Long-Term Outcome

Gonzalez, Lewinsohn, and Clarke (1985) conducted a longitudinal follow-up study of 113 depressed adults who had previously been treated in the Coping with Depression Course to examine 1- to 3-year outcome. The post-treatment recovery rate for adults with major depressive disorder (75%) was significantly higher than the comparable rate for adults with intermittent depression (43%) and adults with "double depression" (27%) (major depression superimposed upon intermittent depression). However, they also found that 54% of those adults who had recovered from their index episode of depression had relapsed within the first 60 weeks after recovery. Thus, only half of recovered patients remained symptom free throughout the follow-up period. For a substantial proportion of patients, the improvement does not constitute a full recovery from the index episode. There were no differences in relapse rates for adults with intermittent or major depression, or adults with primary or secondary depression. That is, even though adults with diagnoses of intermittent and double depression were less likely to recover during treatment, given that a patient had recovered, the relapse rate was not related to diagnosis. Significant predictors of relapse included a greater number of previous episodes of depression, a family history of depression, poor physical health, dissatisfaction with major life roles, higher depression scores at entry into treatment, and younger age. In total, these factors accounted for 38% of the variance in treatment outcome.

Efficacy of the Course with Adolescents

Two studies have examined the efficacy of the Adolescent Coping with Depression Course. The initial study (Clarke, 1985) was conducted with a total of 21 adolescents, 14 of which met Research Diagnostic Criteria (Spitzer, Endicott, and Robins, 1978) for either major depression or intermittent depression at intake. The other 7 adolescents were either exhibiting depressive symptoms that were not intense enough to meet full Research Diagnostic Criteria for diagnosis, or they were identified as depressed by parents and/or teachers but did not report having any depressive symptoms themselves.

The results of this initial study are promising. From intake to post-treatment, the mean BDI score of the treated, clinically depressed adolescents dropped from 15.0 to 4.1 (p<.001). Further, these adolescents did not meet criteria for any affective disorder at the end of treatment, with the exception of one teenager who still met criteria for major depression.

In the second outcome study (Lewinsohn, Clarke, Hops, Andrews, and Williams, 1990), a total of 59 clinically depressed adolescents were randomly assigned to one of three conditions: 1) a cognitive-behavioral, psycho-educational group for adolescents only (N=21); 2) an identical group for adolescents, but with their parents enrolled in a separate group (N=19); and 3) a waiting-list control group (N=19). Adolescents and their parents participated in extensive interviews at intake, post-treatment, and 1- and 6-month follow up. Additional follow-up interviews were conducted at 12- and 24-months post-treatment.

The results of this study are summarized in Tables 2, 3, and 4, and Figure 1. Overall, multivariate analyses demonstrated significant pre- to post-treatment changes in all dependent variables across treatment conditions.

Subsequent planned comparisons indicated that all significant subject improvement was accounted for by the two active treatment conditions. Surprisingly, there were no significant outcome differences between the *Adolescent Only* and the *Adolescent + Parent* treatment conditions on diagnostic and self-report assessments. The only measure that indicated a difference between these two treatment conditions was ratings made by parents on the Child Behavior Checklist (Achenbach, 1978); parents in the *Adolescent + Parent* condition reported significant pre- to post-treatment reductions in problem behaviors. More details regarding the findings of this outcome study are provided in Lewinsohn et al. (1990).

Table 2

**Adolescents Meeting Criteria for Any Depressive Disorder[*]
across the Three Conditions at Pre- and Post-Treatment
and at 1- and 6-Month Follow Up**

	Pre-Tx	Post-Tx	1-Month	6-Month
Adolescent + Parent Group	100.0% (19/19)	52.6% (10/19)	26.3% (5/19)	13.3% (2/15)
Adolescent Only Group	100.0% (21/21)	57.1% (12/21)	35.0% (7/20)	20.0% (3/15)
Waiting-list Group	100.0% (19/19)	94.7% (18/19)	—	—

Pre- vs. Post-Treatment:
    Chi-square = 9.41
            df = 2
            p   < .01

[*]DSM-III-R diagnosis of major depression or dysthymia, or RDC diagnosis of minor depression.

Table 3

Pre- and Post-Treatment Means and Standard Deviations
for Adolescent Scores on the CES-D and BDI
across Three Treatment Conditions

Measure	Group	Pre		Post	
		M	SD	M	SD
CES-D[*]	Adol. Only	13.28	5.20	7.19	4.88
	Adol. + Parent	12.84	6.65	5.68	4.78
	Waiting List	14.89	4.30	12.89	4.74
BDI	Adol. Only	21.66	11.34	10.00	11.91
	Adol. + Parent	21.26	11.35	6.47	8.53
	Waiting List	23.84	11.43	20.47	10.28

[*]Based on a seven-item scale.

Table 4

Means and Standard Deviations for Adolescent
Scores at 1- and 6-Month Follow Up

Measure	Group	Follow Up			
		1-Month		6-Month[*]	
		M	SD	M	SD
CES-D[**]	Adol. Only	6.76	5.34	6.25	4.54
	Adol. + Parent	5.53	4.03	5.41	3.81
BDI	Adol. Only	9.95	11.18	8.23	11.21
	Adol. + Parent	6.68	7.89	6.46	9.51

[*]The mean for each measure was substituted for missing 6-month follow-up data for five Adolescent Only subjects and five Adolescent and Parent subjects.

[**]Based on a seven-item scale.

Figure 1

**Mean BDI Score and Percent Meeting Criteria
for a Diagnosis of Depression from
Intake to 24 Months Post-Treatment**

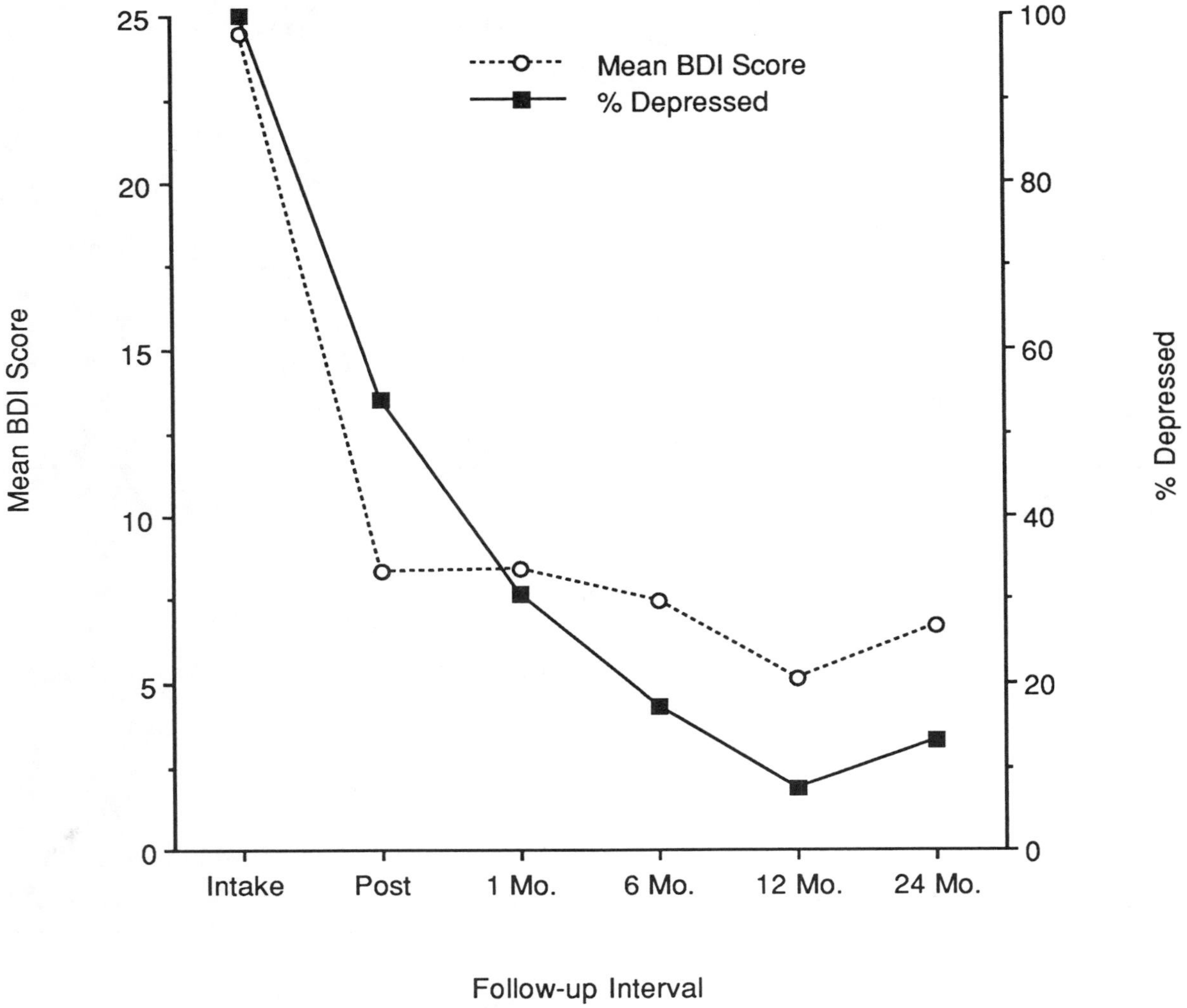

Long-Term Outcome

Because the waiting-list subjects were given an opportunity to participate in the Adolescent Coping with Depression Course immediately following the post-treatment interview, follow-up data for the control condition are not available. For the two active treatment conditions, data were obtained at 1, 6, 12 and 24 months; however, data were missing for approximately half of the adolescents at the 12- and 24-month assessments. Two separate 2 x 4 (Group x Time) multivariate analyses of variance with repeated measures on the second factor (Time) were employed to investigate the maintenance of treatment effects. As indicated in Table 4 and Figure 1, the diagnoses and depression scores remained at very low levels throughout the entire follow-up interval.

CHAPTER 8
Future Directions

Although a considerable amount of research has been conducted on the Adolescent Coping with Depression Course, there are a still number of issues that need to be addressed in future research studies. Some of these issues have been mentioned in previous chapters, but they will be considered again in this chapter in more detail and from a slightly different perspective.

In reviewing the available literature on the Adolescent Coping with Depression Course, it is apparent that the course has been shown to be an effective treatment for unipolar depression when it is used with diagnostically homogeneous populations of depressed adolescents. The amount of improvement and the relapse rate are comparable to those obtained for cognitive-behavioral interventions with adults. Most participants are improved at the end of treatment, and these gains are maintained at 1-, 6-, 12-, and 24-month follow ups. Given the success of the clinical research program to date, it seems appropriate to consider directions for future investigations of the course.

Cross-Validation

It is essential to cross-validate the data on the efficacy of the course. The results obtained by our group need to be replicated in other research settings by other investigators. Perhaps more importantly, replications must be carried out in *real-life* clinical settings. To date, investigations of the course have employed exclusion criteria such that subjects whose depression is co-morbid with drug/alcohol abuse or dependence, conduct disorder, or schizophrenia were excluded. Thus, it is unknown how effective the course will be for dual diagnosis populations. This is a particularly important issue in that several epidemiological studies of adolescent and adult depressives indicate that co-morbidity is high, especially with substance use disorders (e.g., Lewinsohn, Hops, Roberts, and Seeley, 1989). Studies of the course in clinical settings will address the critical issue of external validity; that is, do our findings generalize to clinical settings?

Beyond cross-validation, research is needed to: 1) evaluate the relative importance of specific components of the course and the mechanisms of change; 2) delineate the characteristics of depressed individuals who do not respond to the course and who might respond to other treatments; 3) compare the efficacy of the course with other interventions, both pharmacological and psychotherapeutic; 4) design and evaluate modifications of the course for use with populations that are different from those that have been studied so far; and 5) evaluate the efficacy of the course for prevention.

Mechanisms of Change and Critical Components

One important question concerns the incremental value of including the parents in the treatment program. While the results of our outcome studies to date tend to favor the adolescent plus parent conditions, the effect has been small in magnitude and has failed to attain statistical significance (Lewinsohn, Clarke, Hops, Andrews, and Williams, 1990). We are currently evaluating a modified version of the Adolescent Coping with Depression Course in which the Parent Group is given more attention to ascertain whether this will enhance the impact of parent involvement on treatment outcome. Another important question concerns the relationship between changes in the behaviors that are targeted for modification as a function of treatment and therapeutic change (i.e., depression reduction). This issue has been addressed in several studies (e.g., Zeiss, Lewinsohn, and Muñoz, 1979; Simons, Garfield, and Murphy, 1984) which have shown that comparable changes in various depression-related target behaviors occur in cognitive-behavioral treatment independent of the specific behaviors targeted for intervention (this is also discussed in Chapter 6).

The results of these studies suggest, but do not prove, that change in *specific* target behaviors is not critical for therapeutic change. Yet, there is also evidence that matching specific treatment techniques to patients with particular target problems can produce particular benefits. McKnight, Nelson, Hayes, and Jarrett (1984) found that adult patients with social skills difficulties and irrational cognitions improved more after receiving specific interventions for those deficits than with interventions not related to their presenting problem areas. Conversely, Simons, Lustman, Wetzel, and Murphy (1985) showed that patients who scored high (indicating proficiency) on a measure of learned resourcefulness (Rosenbaum, 1980) showed more improvement in cognitive therapy than in pharmacotherapy. The results of some of these studies (e.g., McKnight et al., 1984) suggest that it may be clinically productive to match treatment components to areas of weakness (compensation model), while others (e.g., Simons et al., 1985) suggest that it is important to match treatment components to areas of strength (capitalization model). The mixed results of these studies raise many important theoretical questions, which have been most clearly explicated by Hollon, Evans, and DeRubeis (1987) and by Rude and Rehm (1989). Future investigations of the Adolescent Coping with Depression Course might examine the relative merits of these two competing models as they relate to mechanisms of change in the cognitive-behavioral treatment of adolescents.

Characteristics of Adolescents Who Do Not Respond to the Course

While our research on the course indicates that most participants improved, approximately 20% failed to respond to treatment. The fact that this figure is consistent with research on failure rates for other treatments of depression (e.g., McLean and Hakstian, 1979; Weissman and Klerman, 1977; Weissman, Klerman, Prusoff, Sholomskas, and Padian, 1981) does not mean that this important subgroup of depressed individuals should be ignored. The studies on treatment outcome for the adult course suggest that patients who did not expect to be improved at the end of treatment, who were dissatisfied with major life roles, who perceived their family environments to be unsupportive, who did not show early positive perceptions of group cohesiveness, and whose pre-treatment depression levels were high were the least improved at the end of treatment (Hoberman, Lewinsohn, and Tilson, 1988). We are in the process of evaluating these predictors of outcome with adolescents. Preliminary results (Clarke, Hops, Lewinsohn, and Andrews, 1990) indicate that three pre-treatment variables significantly accounted for 40% of the variance in treatment outcome ($p = .0002$): positive treatment outcome was associated with: 1) more pessimistic attitudes, 2) greater frequency and higher enjoyability of pleasant events, and 3) more parent-reported conflicts with their adolescents. These results are somewhat surprising, in that they are only partially consistent with results observed among treated adults (e.g., Steinmetz, Breckenridge, Thompson, and Gallagher, 1983; Hoberman et al., 1988).

The results of studies on characteristics of adolescents who respond poorly to the course may have implications for modifications aimed at enhancing the *long-term* efficacy of the course. Perhaps it would be useful to allow additional sessions so that participants can practice specific skills. A number of researchers have advocated allowing more time for the acquisition of specific skills in order to enhance treatment gains and to reduce the likelihood of relapse (e.g., Hollon and Beck, 1987). In the same vein, the use of booster sessions following the end of active treatment may help participants to maintain their gains.

Hollon (1984) has distinguished between two types of predictive information. *Prognostic* information is used to predict which participants will do well in a particular treatment. The studies mentioned earlier on individual predictors of outcome for the adult course shed some light on this area. In contrast, *prescriptive* information addresses the question of which of several treatments will work best for a patient with particular characteristics. Until comparative outcome studies are conducted with the Adolescent Coping with Depression Course, it is not possible to determine which individuals are most appropriate for this type of treatment relative to other modalities. Moreover, such studies might provide theoretically and clinically useful information regarding the specificity of the effects produced by the course. It also may be important to explore the effectiveness of the course when it is used in conjunction with antidepressant medications.

Efficacy of the Course Compared with Other Treatments

Further research is also needed to compare the short- and long-term efficacy of the Adolescent Coping with Depression Course with other treatment alternatives, including pharmacotherapy. While the course is more effective than no treatment, its effectiveness relative to other cognitive-behavioral treatments or to medication is unknown. If the course were to be tested in a comparative outcome study, it would be possible to identify the characteristics of adolescents who would respond better to other treatments. Certainly, pharmacotherapy has been shown to be an effective treatment for unipolar depression among adults. For example, in their review of the literature on imipramine, Klein, Gittelman, Quitkin, and Rifkin (1980) found that 70% of 734 adult patients treated with imipramine improved, compared to 39% of 606 placebo-treated patients. Given the similarities in core symptomology among child, adolescent, and adult depression, it is reasonable to hypothesize similar responses to antidepressant medication.

However, the preliminary data regarding the use of these medications with depressed children and adolescents is somewhat mixed. While a number of initial reports and uncontrolled single-group trials yielded positive results (e.g., Preskorn, Weller, and Weller, 1982), subsequent double-blind placebo-controlled drug trials with depressed children and adolescents suggest that tricyclic antidepressants such as imipramine and amitriptyline are no more effective than a placebo (Ryan et al., 1985; Simeon, Ferguson, Copping, and DiNicola, 1988; Kramer and Feiguine, 1981; Puig-Antich et al., 1987). One of the complications of using these drugs with children and adolescents is that effective dosages are often close to levels at which side effects such as cardiotoxicity, tremors, etc., are first observed (Blau, 1978; Rancurello, 1985).

While future investigation may lead to the development of safe and effective pharmacotherapy for depressed adolescents and children, the unresolved questions regarding the efficacy and safety of antidepressant medication suggest that other treatment modalities should be explored for these populations.

Modifications for Use with Other Populations

The efficacy of the course with dual diagnosis populations is unknown because the exclusion criteria employed in all of our studies did not allow depressed subjects to participate if there was evidence of concurrent schizophrenia, conduct disorder, chemical dependence, or other psychiatric disorders. As indicated earlier, depression is often co-morbid with other disorders. It is likely that patients whose depression is co-morbid with these other disorders may pose new challenges to treatment that will require modifications of the course.

One specific example is the efficacy of the course as an adjunct to the treatment of adolescent substance abuse. Turner, Wehl, Cannon, and Craig (1980) have obtained encouraging results with the behavioral treatment of depression in adult alcoholics using techniques similar to those employed in the Coping with Depression Course.

The course could be tested with hospitalized or institutionalized adolescents. Following the pilot study of Antonuccio, Akins, Chatham, Monagin, Tearnan, and Ziegler (1983), the course could prove to be an effective intervention for hospitalized and/or severely depressed patients as an adjunct to the other treatments that are typically offered to such patients.

Patients with chronic and disabling physical illnesses which require major changes in lifestyle often suffer from depression (Schulberg, McClelland, and Burns, 1987). In adolescents, such diseases or disabilities would include diabetes, epilepsy, injuries, cancer, and chronic fatigue syndrome. The nonstigmatizing nature of the course would make it an appealing intervention for teenagers who do not view their condition as primarily psychiatric. For example, the treatment could be called a "Coping with Diabetes" course, etc. In addition, parents who provide care for chronically ill or disabled adolescents may be at risk for depression themselves, and might also be appropriate candidates for an interventions such as the Coping with Depression Course.

A largely overlooked direction for future research involves populations other than "mainstream" middle class, white Americans. Only a few studies have systematically employed the Coping with Depression Course with cultural or ethnic minority adults (Manson, Mosely, and Brenneman, 1988; Muñoz et al., 1987, 1988). To our knowledge, there have been no studies that have investigated the efficacy of the course as an intervention for minority children or adolescents.

The Prevention of Depression

Most of our work to date has been in what is called tertiary prevention. We have worked with people who are already depressed in an effort to reduce or eliminate their depression and increase the likelihood that they will remain depression-free after treatment. Our results with both adolescent and adult populations have been encouraging. What remains to be tested, however, is the efficacy of the course as a primary or secondary prevention program.

It has become the tradition to define unipolar depression as an episodic, all-or-none disorder. If depression is defined in this way, then the objective of prevention is to reduce incidence—that is, the number of people who develop an episode of depression during a given period of time. However, in evaluating the potential usefulness and effectiveness of any intervention for preventing depression, it is important to realize that depression can just as easily be conceptualized as a continuum. The continuum view of depression involves at least two dimensions: 1) *the severity level*, which reflects the number, frequency, and degree of severity of the symptoms; and 2) *the duration*, which is an indication of how long the symptoms persist. As demonstrated in two previous investigations (Lewinsohn, Fenn, Stanton, and Franklin, 1986; Lewinsohn, Hops, Roberts, and Seeley, 1989), the length of depressive episodes are highly skewed, with most adults and adolescents having relatively short episodes.

This conceptualization of depression as a continuum makes it possible to define somewhat more modest but perhaps more attainable goals for prevention, that is, to reduce the severity and duration of symptoms. In other words, instead of evaluating a given intervention simply in terms of the degree to which it prevents a depressive episode *per se*, an intervention might also have an important preventive function to the extent that it results in episodes that are relatively mild and short-lived (instead of episodes that are more severe and potentially chronic). An intervention capable of doing this would be useful because mild episodes have a much better prognosis (Steinmetz, Lewinsohn, and Antonuccio, 1983; Keller, Shapiro, Lavori, and Wolfe, 1982). In addition, people who are mildly depressed are much less incapacitated in the sense that they can continue to function in important life roles.

We believe that the greatest potential for both the adult and adolescent versions of the Coping with Depression Course in terms of prevention is that it can be used to teach people how to end episodes of depression quickly before they become severe. There is some evidence that supports this assumption.

The adult course has been studied as a means of preventing episodes of depression among individuals presumed to be at elevated risk for developing such episodes. Muñoz, Ying, Armas, Chan, and Gurza (1987) modified the course and employed it with a group known to be at high risk for future depressive disorders: low income, minority, adult medical outpatients. Persons already experiencing an episode of depression were excluded from the study. Members of the experimental group were compared to two control groups: a no-intervention group and an information-only group (e.g., they received a 40-minute videotape presentation of the ideas in the course). Subjects were randomly assigned to the different groups. The modified course consisted of eight 2-hour sessions. Follow-up rates at one year were 92%. The results indicated that the subjects who participated in the course showed a significantly greater decrease in the level of depressive symptoms as measured by the BDI (Muñoz, Ying, Bernal, Perez-Stable, Sorensen, and Hargreaves, 1988). At the 1-year follow-up, none of the individuals who participated in the course experienced a major depressive episode, in contrast to 2/25 of subjects who dropped out of treatment and 4/72 of the controls.

Most recently, Manson and colleagues (Manson, Moseley, and Brenneman, 1988; Manson, 1988) have modified the Coping with Depression Course for use as a prevention intervention with American Indians 45 years of age and older. Participants were at high risk for depression and other psychological disorders because they were having difficulties coping with stressors and there were deficits associated with chronic physical illnesses. The course was modified to make it culturally relevant for the tribes from three northwest reservations, and it was simplified to accommodate the limitations imposed by the physical illnesses of the participants. The specific aim of this modified course was to teach participants coping skills and strategies *in advance* of failure to cope.

An intervention trial of this preventive modification of the course is currently underway. The participants are 60 tribal residents of three northwest reservations with a recent diagnosis of a deteriorating physical health condition (e.g., diabetes, rheumatoid arthritis, etc.). Participants have been randomly assigned to either the prevention group or to a waiting-list control condition. Intake and post-intervention interviews are currently being conducted, and follow-up evaluations will also be conducted at 6 and 12 months.

Further research evaluating the preventive function of the Coping with Depression Course with other populations known to be at elevated risk for depression appears warranted. On the basis of several epidemiological studies (Hirschfeld and Cross, 1982; Lewinsohn, Hoberman, and Rosenbaum, 1988), information that can be used to select at-risk populations is rapidly becoming available. We now know that the following groups are at elevated risk for episodes of depression: 1) women, 2) people who have experienced previous episodes of depression, 3) individuals who are mildly depressed, 4) people with weak social support systems, 5) the unemployed and those seeking employment, 6) persons involved in marital conflict, and 7) individuals who have experienced recent stressful life events, especially those involving social exits (e.g., divorce and separation).

Individuals afflicted with medical illnesses or disabilities which require major changes in their lifestyles, but who are not yet depressed, might also benefit from the coping skills taught in the course. The course may serve a similar preventive function for patients who are in remission from other disorders (e.g., alcoholism) and are at elevated risk for depression. Finally, there is a large group of individuals who are mildly depressed or dysphoric, a group that Frank (1974) described as "demoralized." Such persons manifest symptoms but do not meet full criteria for a diagnosis of depression. Research has demonstrated that these demoralized individuals are at high risk for developing an episode of depression (Lewinsohn, Hoberman, and Rosenbaum, 1988). By teaching skills to reduce dysphoria, the course would serve a significant preventive function if it resulted in episodes of depression that were relatively mild and short-lived instead of more severe and potentially chronic episodes.

The discussion so far has focused on past and future prevention research with adults. Similarly, the efficacy of the Adolescent Coping with Depression Course as a preventive program warrants further research as well. The course might serve a useful preventive function with adolescents who are known to be at elevated risk for depression. The target groups would include children of depressed parents (e.g., Weissman et al., 1987), teenagers who are already mildly depressed or dysphoric, pregnant adolescents (Goldklang, 1989), teenagers recovering from chemical dependency, teenagers who have recently moved or lost a parent through divorce or death, and adolescents with chronic illness or disabilities.

At a general preventive level, the Adolescent Coping with Depression Course could be offered as a "life skills" course in high schools, perhaps as part of a health curriculum. It seems reasonable to assume that the skills taught in the course are appropriate for nondepressed as well as depressed individuals. In such a mass approach, all adolescents could learn how to recognize early manifestations of depression and what to do to minimize the impact in their lives. The skills taught in the course can also be used to deal with stress, develop self-control, and improve interpersonal functioning, although the hypothesis that adolescents would benefit from these skills has not been tested.

Given the increasing knowledge of the various populations at risk for depression and the apparent robust flexibility of the adult and adolescent versions of the Coping with Depression Course, research examining the preventive function of the course with these groups promises to be fruitful.

SECTION II
Course Sessions

This section provides a detailed outline of the 16 sessions that comprise the Adolescent Coping with Depression Course. The sessions are highly structured and follow a rigorous agenda. It is essential for group leaders to become familiar with the format, content, and pace of the course before attempting to conduct the sessions. The first step is to read through all of the sessions to develop a grasp of the various content areas and the progression of the material. It is also assumed that group leaders have read at least the first six chapters in Section I.

Several different methods of instruction are employed in the course to help the adolescents learn new material: lectures by the group leader, discussions, demonstration activities, group activities, team activities, role-playing exercises, and homework assignments. The following format conventions indicate the method of presentation:

The text that is meant to be read out loud as a lecture is indented and appears in bold type. Of course, leaders are welcome to change the lectures at their own discretion as they become more comfortable with the various content areas.

Leader: This tag is used to identify directions for the group leader. The text is set in regular type.

Group Activity

Large headings mark the beginning of the various activities.

| WORKBOOK | This is a signal that students need to turn to a specific page in their workbooks. |

This box appears at the beginning of each session as a reminder to bring materials:

Materials needed for this session:

Text for the group leader to write on the blackboard is highlighted in this manner:

BLACKBOARD

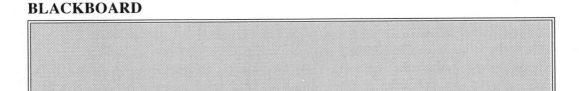

It should also be noted that there are two different versions of Sessions 12, 13, and 14. The version that is included with the rest of the course sessions is intended for use with "Adolescent Only" groups. When parents are not involved in the program, the students practice the problem-solving and negotiation skills presented in Sessions 13 and 14 by role playing with one another. Then, as part of their homework assignment, they work on the same skills with their parents. The other version of these sessions, which appear in Section III, are used when parents participate in the program by attending a separate group that is specifically designed for them (a *Leader's Manual for Parent Groups* and a *Parent Workbook* are available from the publisher). During Sessions 13 and 14, the groups for parents and adolescents are joined together and each family takes turns applying the problem-solving and negotiation skills.

The group leader should always arrive 10 minutes early to set up the room and write the agenda on the blackboard. If there is sufficient time, the leader should begin the session with a brief oral review of the agenda. It may be necessary to skip this review for some of the sessions in which there is an inordinate amount of material to cover and time is short.

SESSION 1
Depression and Social Learning

Materials needed for this session:
1. Workbooks for all adolescents.
2. Extra pens and pencils.
3. Refreshments for the break.

<u>Leader</u>: Write the Agenda and Rule on the blackboard at the beginning of each class session.

BLACKBOARD

AGENDA
    I.   MOOD QUESTIONNAIRE (10 min.)
    II.   GUIDELINES FOR THIS CLASS (10 min.)
   III. GET-ACQUAINTED ACTIVITY (40 min.)
        Break (10 min.)
    IV. HOW TO CHANGE YOUR LIFE (25 min.)
    V.   MOOD DIARY (10 min.)
   VI. HOMEWORK ASSIGNMENT (10 min.)
  VII. QUIZ (5 min.)

RULE: People like you if you like them.

Introductions

<u>Leader</u>: Briefly introduce yourself and get the names of participants. Save lengthier introductions for the Get-Acquainted Activity.

I. MOOD QUESTIONNAIRE (10 min.)

WORKBOOK

Ask students to turn to the "Beginning of the Course" Mood Questionnaire provided in the Appendix of their workbooks.

In this class we're going to learn some ways to control the way we feel. Before we start, we need to measure how you feel about yourself and your life now. At the end of the course, we will again measure how you feel to see how much improvement there is. I want everyone to fill out the Mood Questionnaire right now. I will be the only one reading your responses, so please answer the questions honestly.

<u>Leader</u>: After everyone has finished, give instructions for scoring.

To score the questionnaire, add up all of the numbers you have circled. If you have circled more than one number for a statement, add only the highest number to your score. You may notice that the numbers for your responses on four of the statements (#4, #8, #12, and #16) are listed in reverse order. This has been done on purpose, and your score will be correct if you simply add up the numbers you have circled.

<u>Leader</u>: Collect the completed Mood Questionnaires from the students; check the scores and record them after the session. Return the Mood Questionnaires to students during the next session.

II. GUIDELINES FOR THIS CLASS (10 min.)

WORKBOOK

Ask students to turn to page 1.3 in their workbooks.

The following are some rules that must be observed in this course so we can help each other:

1. *AVOID DEPRESSIVE TALK.* Use the group for support, but not as a sounding board for your depression. The best support comes from helping each other get away from depressive talk. We want to focus on positive changes.

2. *ALLOW EACH PERSON TO HAVE EQUAL TIME.* To get the most from the course, each of you should have an opportunity to share ideas, ask questions, and discuss any difficulties you have in using the techniques.

3. *THE PERSONAL THINGS WE TALK ABOUT IN CLASS ARE NOT TO BE SHARED OUTSIDE THIS GROUP.*
   a. Any information discussed in the intake interview will remain confidential and will not be shared with the group.
   b. Everyone is expected to honor the confidentiality rule by not discussing personal material from their group sessions with people who aren't part of the group. Of course, there is always the possibility that someone will violate this rule; if any of you have concerns about confidentiality, please feel free to talk to me about it.

4. *OFFER SUPPORT.* Your comments and feedback should be:
   a. *CONSTRUCTIVE.* Avoid criticism; "zapping" and sarcasm aren't allowed.
   b. *REWARDING.* Focus on the positive aspects of what others are doing or saying, and build on that with praise and approval.
   c. *CARING.* Show the other members of your group that you care about them by being thoughtful and respectful.
   d. *NONPRESSURING.* Don't force others to do something they don't want to do.

Remember—we all have something to contribute, so let's try to help one another.

III. GET-ACQUAINTED ACTIVITY (40 min.)

Objectives
1. To discuss the idea that learning to control your life is a skill.
2. To present four criteria for a positive social interaction and to help each student identify the things he or she does well.
3. To help each student select one friendly skill to work on.

Learning to Control Your Life

Who or what controls your life?

Leader: Ask students to volunteer some answers to this question. Write their suggestions on the blackboard. Modify the following dialogue to fit the suggestions offered. If the responses focus on external factors, write a big *YOU* on the blackboard under them. If some of the answers indicate the self is in control, circle them. Typically, the students will focus on external factors instead of asserting that they are in control of their own lives to any great extent.

There are many factors controlling your life, but the one we want to focus on is *YOU*. You *can* control many aspects of your life, even if you don't right now. You can learn to control how you feel and improve your mood. Most of the teenagers entering this course feel they have little or no control over their moods. In this course you will learn *SKILLS* that will help you overcome feelings of depression, and you will find that with these skills you can, indeed, control your mood.

BLACKBOARD

RULE: Learning to control your life is a skill. You will be learning skills for controlling your life in this class.

What do you have to do to learn a new skill? For example, playing the piano is a skill. What do you have to do to learn to play the piano?

PRACTICE is an important part of this class. You will be given new skills in class, and you will need to practice them every day. This daily practice is your "homework."

The first skill we are going to practice is *MEETING PEOPLE*. Starting a conversation is one way to show people that you like them, and it gives them a chance to show that they like you, too. Liking people and being liked makes us happier. The rule for this session is that people like you if you like them.

Making Interactions with New People Positive

How do you show people that you are a friendly person?

<u>Leader</u>: Solicit answers from students. Give everyone a chance to offer suggestions. Then summarize their ideas and examples as you list the following criteria on the blackboard. You may want to change the order so that you add the ideas they didn't mention last.

How to be a friendly person:
1. **Look at the person's eyes when you are talking or listening.**
2. **Smile at least once, the more often the better.**
3. **Say something positive about the other person.**
4. **Tell about yourself.**

<u>Leader</u>: Short form to write on the blackboard for easier recall:

BLACKBOARD

> 1. Make eye contact.
> 2. Smile.
> 3. Say positive things.
> 4. Tell about yourself.

| WORKBOOK | Ask students to answer questions #1, #2, and #3 on page 1.4.

Team Activity

We're going to practice doing these things as we get acquainted with each other. You are going to tell about yourself and listen to someone tell about him- or herself. Here are some questions you can use to learn more about each other:

<u>Leader</u>: Write the following questions on the blackboard. Don't erase the "how to be a friendly person" list.

BLACKBOARD

> ## Interview Questions
> 1. Where are you from?
> 2. What are your hobbies?
> 3. What do you do well?
> 4. Who are the important people in your life?
> 5. Do you have any pets?

<u>Leader</u>: Pair off students or form groups of three. The goal in this exercise is for students to learn more about each other; then the students will introduce one another to the rest of the class.

> **Now you and your teammate are going to *TAKE TURNS TELLING ABOUT YOURSELVES*. Remember to use the techniques that make a positive interaction as you do this. When you have finished, you will introduce your teammate to the rest of the class.**

<u>Leader</u>: Model this process by briefly introducing yourself, touching on as many of the interview questions written on the blackboard as possible. As the students participate in the exercise, make sure you reinforce and praise them (particularly the shy and withdrawn adolescents) for their attempts to use the friendly skills and interview questions. Then have students introduce their teammates to the rest of the class. After they have finished, have them give each other constructive feedback by using the procedure outlined below.

Providing Constructive Feedback

> **Stay with the same teammate. Now you're going to be supportive and give each other *CONSTRUCTIVE FEEDBACK* about how friendly each of you were. This is how you do it. First, look at the "How to be a friendly person" list on the blackboard, and comment on the things your teammate *DID WELL*. Then name one thing from the list that your teammate could have done better to look more friendly. Even if two or more things need improvement, just mention the *ONE THING* that would make the most difference. Each person should end up with one thing that he or she could do better. All of us have something we need to work on. Nobody is perfect.**

<u>Leader</u>: Model how to provide constructive feedback. Pick one adolescent, and describe the friendly skills he or she did well first, then name one skill that person could do better.

Ask students to answer and correct questions #4 and #5 on page 1.4.

Your answer to question #5 on page 1.4 is your *FIRST GOAL* in this course, and it is your homework assignment for the next few days. Turn to the Session Goal Record, which is page 1.2 at the front of your workbook, and write "Use friendly skills" on the line for Session 1. Your homework assignment is to have conversations with people you know and to practice the friendly skill you need to work on.

<u>Leader</u>: Model how to practice friendly skills.

Break (10 min.)

You can practice your friendly skills right now while we take a *10-minute* break.

IV. HOW TO CHANGE YOUR LIFE (25 min.)

Objectives
1. To outline for students the three aspects of each individual's personality that contribute to depression.
2. To help each student identify whether a thought, feeling, or action contributes to his or her downward spiral of depression.

Your Personality Is a Three-Part System

Now we're going to talk about how we look at depression. Our perspective is that each of us has a personality that is a three-part system.

<u>Leader</u>: Draw the following diagram on the blackboard. Point out that the diagram also appears at the bottom of page 1.4 in the workbook.

BLACKBOARD

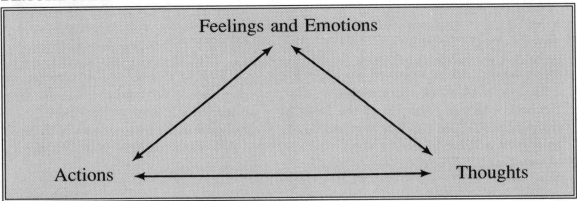

Feelings and Emotions

Actions ← → Thoughts

Depression can start in any of these three areas: feelings and emotions, actions, and thoughts. Each area affects the other two. Which of these parts of ourselves do you think are easiest to control?

<u>Leader</u>: If students focus on changing emotions first, respond by saying, "Most people try to change their emotions; for example, they try to feel better first, but this is the hardest part to change. It is much easier to learn skills to change your thoughts and actions, and this will, in turn, change how you feel."

DEPRESSIVE actions and thoughts have unpleasant and dissatisfying results. POSITIVE actions and thoughts make us feel good.

Which of the following thoughts and actions are DEPRESSIVE, and which are POSITIVE?
1. **Withdrawing from friends.**
2. **Having fun with friends.**
3. **Telling yourself that you are boring.**
4. **Reminding yourself about someone who cares about you.**

| WORKBOOK | Ask students to answer questions #6 through #9 on page 1.5.

<u>Leader</u>: As the students work on the questions, walk around the room giving assistance. When 80% of the students have finished, correct their work. This is a general guideline—don't make the majority wait too long for a few. Give assistance to any stragglers; allow them to fill in answers and make corrections as you go over the answers.

Emotional Spirals

When we feel bad, we're less likely to do things we enjoy, and we then have doubts about our ability to be successful doing those things (for example, making new friends). When we're successful at doing something, we feel good and we gain self-confidence. When we can do something well, we feel good and are encouraged to do more things in the future.

<u>Leader</u>: Draw the following diagrams on the blackboard:

BLACKBOARD

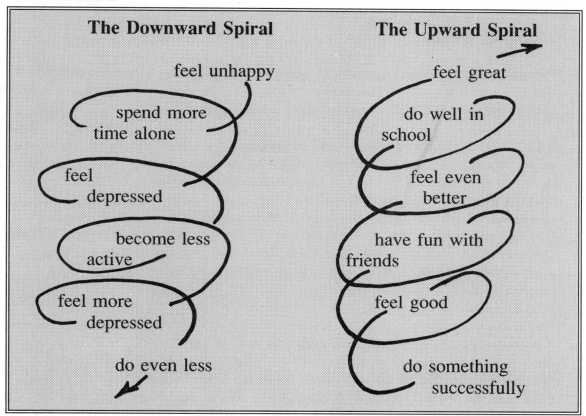

You can think of either of these as *A SPIRAL* that can move in one direction or the other. How you feel affects how you think and behave, which then affects how you feel and think, and so on. Think about the triangle we discussed earlier that represents the three parts of your personality.

These are some of the things that can start a spiral *DOWNWARD* into depression:
1. Participating in few positive or fun activities.
2. Feeling depressed.
3. Doing less.
4. Thinking negative thoughts.
5. Feeling even worse, then doing less, etc.

These are some of the things that can start a spiral *UPWARD*, or get you "on a roll." A positive spiral can break the negative cycle and reverse it.
1. Being successful at something.
2. Feeling confident.
3. Doing more fun things.
4. Having friends.

I'm going to read two examples to you. While you listen to these examples, I want you to think about two things. First, what kind of spiral is represented in each example? Second, what keeps the spiral going?

EXAMPLE 1. Mark, a 16-year-old sophomore, had done poorly at school for many months. He began telling himself that he was a failure and that he would never be successful at anything. Over the course of a few months, he started withdrawing from his friends and spending more time alone in his room, thinking that no one liked him or wanted to spend time with him. He began feeling depressed, down, gloomy, and tired. He also found that he had difficulty concentrating, and his grades got even worse. He started skipping school several days a week, and he spent the days alone, unhappy and confused.

EXAMPLE 2. When Mark began coming to the group, he was sure that things would never get better for him. However, he worked with the group to develop a plan to change the negative thoughts he was telling himself, and to replace those thoughts with more positive self-statements. In the past, Mark had enjoyed playing his guitar with some musician friends, but when he became depressed he stopped doing this altogether. With encouragement from the group, Mark started jamming with his friends again. As Mark became more socially active and spent less time thinking negative thoughts about himself, he found his depression lifting and his mood improving, even though he had done nothing directly to try to change his mood.

Can you give me an example of a downward spiral? How about an example of an upward spiral?

┌─────────────────┐
│ **WORKBOOK** │ Ask students to turn to page 1.6.
└─────────────────┘

Question #10 asks you to think of things that cause a downward spiral for you. List some specific thoughts and actions that make you feel depressed.

<u>Leader</u>: Give an example of a *specific* thought as you describe a downward spiral of your own. Get the students to identify very specific thoughts.

Question #11 asks you to think of things that lead to an upward spiral for you. List some specific thoughts and actions that make you feel better.

<u>Leader</u>: Give an example of a *specific* thought as you describe an upward spiral of your own.

In this course, we are going to learn skills to change the downward spiral to an upward one. We will work on changing *ACTIONS* by:
1. **Increasing pleasant activities—doing more fun things.**
2. **Improving social skills—we have already started doing this by working on a friendly skill.**
3. **Developing effective communication and problem-solving skills.**

We will work on changing *THOUGHTS* by:
1. **Stopping negative thoughts.**
2. **Increasing positive thoughts.**

We will work on changing *FEELINGS* by:
1. **Changing our thoughts.**
2. **Changing our actions.**
3. **Learning relaxation skills.**

V. MOOD DIARY (10 min.)

Objective
1. To show students how to fill out the Mood Diary.

Monitoring How You Feel

```
┌─────────────┐
│ WORKBOOK    │    Ask students to turn to page 1.1.
└─────────────┘
```

Our goal in this course is to change the way we feel. We're going to monitor how we feel throughout the course by filling out a Mood Diary. The Mood Diary uses a *SEVEN-POINT SCALE*. Before we talk about the seven-point scale of the Mood Diary, let's see how you would use a scale like this with other things. On a scale of 1 to 7, how warm are you right now? A rating of 7 is very, very hot, and 1 is very, very cold.

<u>Leader</u>: Try to determine whether the students know how to use a seven-point scale by the way they answer this question. If they seem confused, go through several more examples that are based on information that is relatively objective so you can check the results. The following are some suggestions: How warm is it at the North Pole? How warm is it in the desert? How warm is it in Oregon on the average? How warm is it today (more or less than the average?

If necessary, consider some examples that are based on continuous dimensions such as difficulty, brightness, speed, redness, and so on. Keep doing this until you are sure the students all know how to use a seven-point scale.

Mood Anchors

The seven-point scale of the Mood Diary in your workbook is used in a similar way. It's harder to decide what number our moods should have, however, without something to anchor the numbers to. So think of the *BEST YOU HAVE EVER FELT IN YOUR LIFE*. Write something down in your Mood Diary to remind you of this moment. Now give this mood a number. If you think it's possible for you to feel even better than this, give it a 5.5 or maybe a 6.

<u>Leader</u>: Write an example of a good mood anchor on the blackboard.

Now think of the *WORST YOU HAVE EVER FELT*. Write something down in your Mood Diary to remind you of this moment, and give it a number. If you think it would be impossible for you to feel any worse, give it a 1. If you might be able to feel worse, give it a 2.

<u>Leader</u>: Write an example of a depressed mood anchor on the blackboard.

Now compare how you feel today with these two feelings. Give today's feeling a number, and write the number in the correct box on page 1.1 in your workbook. Then circle the corresponding number above the box.

<u>Leader</u>: Model this process with a personal example.

Tomorrow you can compare how you feel with how you felt today and with your mood anchors. Every day at about this time you should compare how you feel with the worst and best moments of your life and with how you felt the day before, too. Then write a number in the box for that day. *IT'S IMPORTANT TO DO THIS AT THE SAME TIME EVERY DAY.*

VI. HOMEWORK ASSIGNMENT (10 min.)

WORKBOOK   Ask students to turn to the homework assignment on page 1.7.

Notice that the homework assignment for this session is described on page 1.7. Now I want to you to look at the Session Goal Record on page 1.2 in your workbook. This is where you write your goals for the days between each session. Working on these goals will be part of your homework assignment. Your assignment for this session is to do the following.

1. **Work on your session goal, which is to practice the friendly skill you listed on question #5 on page 1.4 in your workbook. Put a checkmark in the box on the right-hand side of the Session Goal Record if you meet your goal.**

2. **Keep track of how you feel by filling out your Mood Diary (page 1.1).**
   a. **How often should you fill out the Mood Diary?**
      (Answer: Every day.)
   b. **What time of the day should you fill it out?**
      (Answer: At about this time.)

<u>Leader</u>: Have students repeat out loud as a group the two things they need to do this week. Then have them write these two things as goals for Session 1 on page 1.2 in the workbook.

3. **And, last but not least, *REMEMBER TO BRING YOUR WORKBOOK TO EVERY SESSION!!***

Are there any questions?

First Day Success

Let's work on your session goal right now. Talk with someone you met tonight, and use your friendly skills. This way, you'll be practicing your first goal.

Preview the Next Session

Next session, we'll learn some ways to control our thoughts and actions.

VII.   QUIZ (5 min.)

| WORKBOOK |

Ask students to take the quiz on depression and social learning on page 1.8.

Leader: After everyone has finished, read the answers out loud and have each student correct his or her own quiz.

IMPORTANT REMINDER: Make sure the Pleasant Events Schedule—Adolescent Version filled out by each student during the intake interview is scored before the next session. Directions for scoring the Pleasant Events Schedule are provided in Appendix 3. (A computerized scoring program is available from the publisher.)

SESSION 1 QUIZ
Depression and Social Learning

1. Your personality is a three-part system. Name the three parts. (Hint: Remember the triangle?)
   a. _Feelings (Emotions)_
   b. _Thoughts_
   c. _Behavior (Actions)_

2. Name the four things we said a friendly person does.
   a. _Make eye contact_
   b. _Smile_
   c. _Say positive things about the other person_
   d. _Tell about yourself_

3. Can people control their feelings?
   (a.) Yes, with practice.
   b. Not at all.

4. Which way is your mood spiral likely to go if you do the following things? Circle "U" or "D" to indicate upward or downward.

	Upward	Downward
Having fun with friends.	(U)	D
Thinking you are stupid.	U	(D)
Believing no one loves you.	U	(D)
Telling someone something you like about them.	(U)	D

5. Is it possible for people to change or control their thoughts? (Yes)   No

SESSION 2
Self-Observation and Change

Materials needed for this session:
1. Extra workbooks (in case students forget theirs).
2. Extra pens and pencils.
3. Refreshments for the break.
4. Mood Questionnaires completed by students during Session 1.
5. A printout of each student's responses on the Pleasant Events Schedule—Adolescent Version.

BLACKBOARD

AGENDA
    I.   HOMEWORK REVIEW (15 min.)
    II. STARTING A CONVERSATION (30 min.)
       Break (10 min.)
    III. HOW TO DO A BASELINE STUDY (15 min.)
    IV. BASELINE STUDY OF PLEASANT ACTIVITIES (35 min.)
    V. HOMEWORK ASSIGNMENT (10 min.)
    VI. QUIZ (5 min.)

RULE: The key to changing is careful self-observation.

I. HOMEWORK REVIEW (15 min.)

<u>Leader</u>: Return the Mood Questionnaires filled out during the last session to the students.

In the last session, we talked about depression as a problem in living. Before I introduce any new material, let's quickly review the points we have already covered. This is an oral quiz. I'm going to ask some questions—if you think you know the answer, please raise your hand.

Oral Review/Quiz

1. **We discussed the idea that your personality is a three-part system. What are the three parts?**
    (Answer: Actions, thoughts, and feelings.)

2. **Which are the two parts that are easiest to control?**
    (Answer: Actions and thoughts.)

3. **Why would we want to control our actions and our thoughts?**
    (Answer: Because they affect our emotions.)

4. **What is a downward emotional spiral?**
    (Answer: Doing and thinking things that make you feel progressively worse.)

5. **What is an upward emotional spiral?**
    (Answer: Doing and thinking things that make you feel progressively better.)

6. **Can we control a downward spiral and change it into a positive one?**
    (Answer: Yes.)

7. **What are the four things we can do to be a friendly person?**
    (Answer: Have eye contact, smile, say positive things about the other person, and tell about yourself.)

8. **What is the one thing we want to change in this course?**
    (Answer: How we feel.)

9. **How do we keep track of the way we feel?**
   (Answer: By filling out the Mood Diary on page 1.1.)

Review Student Progress/Record Forms

A. **Session Goal (page 1.2)**

1. **Did you think about the friendly skill you were supposed to practice when you talked with people during the last several days?**
2. **Did you practice the friendly skill and record this on your Session Goal Record (page 1.2)?**

Leader: Reward or praise those who practiced a friendly skill (for example, with a handshake, some Hershey's Chocolate Kisses, etc.).

3. **Do you feel that the practice helped?**
4. **Did you find that people responded more positively when you were working on being a friendly person?**
5. **Is it true that people like you if you like them?**

B. **Mood Monitoring (page 1.1)**

1. **How did you remind yourself to fill out your Mood Diary?**
2. **Did you have any problems assigning a number to your mood?**
3. **If your mood fluctuated, did you remember to take the average?**
4. **If you forgot to rate your mood on a particular day, try to remember how you felt, and fill in the number. Remember, though, the ratings are much more accurate if you make them on a daily basis.**

II. STARTING A CONVERSATION (30 min.)

Objectives
1. To help students recognize appropriate times to start a conversation.
2. To give feedback as students identify and generate good and bad "conversation-starter" questions.
3. To have each student write several original questions for starting a conversation with people in the room.
4. To involve students in a role-playing exercise in which they practice starting a conversation in an appropriate situation.

In this course, we're going to spend some time talking about (and practicing) what we call *SOCIAL SKILLS*. These are behaviors that we all use to get along with people. What are some examples of social skills?

<u>Leader</u>: Write the suggestions offered by students on the blackboard. If necessary, add some of the following to the list: making friends, being a good listener, introducing yourself to new people, getting your point across to other people, solving problems without fighting, etc.

Although most of you already know how to do many of these things, we will still *PRACTICE* them in this class. The reason for this is that when people are depressed, they sometimes stop using their social skills altogether and withdraw from people, or they start using inappropriate responses and begin having more fights, talking negatively, or being rude, even though they used to have better skills.

Even if this doesn't apply to you, we still want each of you to practice social skills in this class. Everyone can benefit from a little practice—it's a good way to receive constructive feedback from others, and you will get to know each other in the process. The feedback will help you notice the good things you already do, and it will also point out some areas that need improvement.

Guidelines for Starting Conversations

One of the hardest things for most people to do is to start a conversation. In general, people are afraid of being rejected or looking foolish, although realistically this seldom happens. The two main issues are *WHEN TO START A CONVERSATION* and *WHAT TO SAY*.

Identifying Appropriate Times to Start a Conversation

I'm going to describe a person in several different situations, and I want you to tell me whether these would be appropriate or inappropriate times for you to start a conversation with this person.

<u>Leader</u>: Write the headings *APPROPRIATE* and *INAPPROPRIATE* on the blackboard.

The following are some sample situations you can use for this exercise. As students identify whether a given situation is an appropriate or inappropriate time to start a conversation, list the situations under the corresponding heading on the blackboard. Once the students understand how the exercise works, ask them to suggest some examples; do this as soon as you can. Continue supplying examples until you get some contributions from the students.

Sample Situations
>   **The person makes eye contact.**
>   **The person looks busy.**
>   **The person says "Hello."**
>   **The person looks preoccupied.**
>   **The person looks angry.**
>   **You are in a common situation (waiting for a bus, etc.).**

<u>Leader</u>: The blackboard should look like this when you are finished:

BLACKBOARD

Appropriate	Inappropriate
The person makes eye contact.	The person looks busy.
The person says "Hello."	The person looks preoccupied.
You are in a common situation.	The person looks angry.

In addition to recognizing these signals from other people, you can use them to let people know that *YOU* are willing to start a conversation. How could you use these signals to let someone know that you are willing to start a conversation?
(Answer: Make eye contact, say "Hello," etc.)

Demonstration Exercise

<u>Leader</u>: Act out the situations described above, asking students whether this is an appropriate time to start a conversation. Begin with clearly appropriate and inappropriate pairs of situations. For example, in situation one, look very busy, and in situation two, look idle. End the exercise with pairs that are only minimally different. For example, in situation one, look preoccupied, but make eye contact; and in situation two, look preoccupied, and don't make eye contact.

WORKBOOK	Ask students to answer and correct question #1 on page 2.1.

Good Questions for Starting Conversations

Questions that have more than one word answers are best for starting conversations and keeping them going. The idea is to get the other person to talk about him- or herself.

Let's think of some good and bad conversation-starter questions.

Are these good questions?
1. What time is it?
2. What kinds of cars do you like?
3. Why do you like him/her?
4. Did you know you have a rip in your pants?
5. What's a good way to cool off in this heat?
6. What kind of music do you like?

What kinds of questions can you think of?

Leader: Encourage humor. Write the students' suggestions on the blackboard.

Ask students to answer and correct question #2 on page 2.1. Have students reword the questions that need improvement.

The best opening lines for conversations are often found in the immediate situation. Observe the situation carefully to find topics for conversations.

Demonstration Exercise

Leader: Model using "conversation-starter" questions with some students in the group. Base the questions on things you have observed about them.

Ask students to answer and correct question #3 on page 2.1. Encourage them to generate at least three questions they could use to start a conversation.

Cumulative Practice

In the following situations, decide whether you should start a conversation, and think of questions you could use to initiate the conversation:

1. **What could you say to someone who is reading a fishing magazine on the bus?**
   (Answer: You probably shouldn't bother the person unless he or she stops reading.)

2. **What could you say to start a conversation with someone at a party who is wearing a Cascade-Run-Off (or Butte-to-Butte) T-shirt?**
   (Answer: "Did you run the Cascade last year?" Then follow up with questions about running.)

3. **What could you say to someone who speaks with a strange accent?**
   (Answer: Ask them where they are from, are they visiting, etc.)

4. **Other specific examples.**

<u>Leader</u>: Again, encourage students to come up with some hypothetical situations, and generate possible conversation-starter questions.

Demonstration Exercise

<u>Leader</u>: Role play inappropriate then appropriate conversation starting with students, where you initiate the conversation. If possible, make the incorrect role plays humorous and general. Ask students to identify whether the conversation starting was appropriate or inappropriate.

Would anyone else like to try?

<u>Leader</u>: Assume the part of the "stranger," and let the student volunteers try to start a conversation. They must decide if it is appropriate to start a conversation, then ask an appropriate conversation-starter question. Keep the role plays brief—a maximum of about *1 minute* each.

ROLE-PLAY SUGGESTIONS. The students will probably be very shy about volunteering to participate in this role-playing exercise. The best approach is to be matter-of-fact about it; indicate that you expect everyone to take part in the role-playing exercises throughout the course. Other suggestions for dealing with resistance to role playing include: (a) having the whole group do the first few role plays together so no one feels that he or she is on the spot; (b) having the students or leader role play the wrong way first, then the right way; (c) praising all efforts to role play, and focusing on the positive aspects when giving feedback; (d) using humor and funny situations; and (e) having students use the scripted "personalities" on page 2.8 in their workbooks for the first few role plays.

| WORKBOOK | Ask students to turn to the Session Goal Record on page 1.2. |

The goal for Session 2 is to start a conversation with someone at least twice before the next session. Write "Start two conversations" on the line for Session 2. Put a checkmark in the box if you reach your goal.

Break (10 min.)

You can practice starting conversations right now while we take a *10-minute* break.

III. HOW TO DO A BASELINE STUDY (15 min.)

Objectives
1. To demonstrate how to do a simple baseline count.
2. To help students understand how to look for and interpret patterns in baseline charts.

Leader: Underline the rule on the blackboard as you read it out loud, "The key to changing is careful self-observation."

For every downward emotional spiral, there's an upward one. The key to changing a downward spiral to an upward one is to observe exactly what we do or think that may cause the spiral. The technique we use for identifying what we need to change is called *BASELINING*. Baselining means counting something specific.

Instructions for Doing a Simple Baseline Count

You can do a baseline count on almost anything. To illustrate how this works, I want you to count how often something happens from now to the end of the session. The behavior I want you to observe is how often you contribute something in class.

| WORKBOOK | Ask students to turn to page 2.2. |

At the top of page 2.2, make a slash mark like this [model how this is done] **every time you say something, answer a question, or otherwise contribute to the class. While you do that, I will count the number of times I ask a question. I will make my slash marks on the blackboard.**

Why Is Baselining Important?

During the next few weeks, we will be baselining different aspects of our personalities: our activities, our thoughts, our social interactions, and our relaxation levels. Baselining is very helpful because it gives us *INFORMATION*. We can use this information to *SET GOALS* that will change the way we are. The rule for this session is that the key to changing is careful self-observation. Our first baseline study will focus on the number of *PLEASANT ACTIVITIES* we engage in.

At the bottom of page 2.2 there is a chart of the baseline information Susan recorded in her Mood Diary and daily totals of pleasant activities (page 2.4). When we look at this chart, we need to ask ourselves the two questions listed at the top of the page. Let's look at the first question.

1. **Do mood and pleasant activities relate?**

<u>Leader</u>: Remember to make a slash mark on the blackboard when you ask a question.

Look at Susan's chart. The dashed line is her daily mood score, and the solid line is the daily total of pleasant activities. See how both lines tend to move up and down together? This means that one probably causes the other.
   a. **Is Susan's mood related to the number of pleasant activities she does?**
      (Answer: Yes, mood and the number of pleasant activities are usually closely related.)
   b. **When we're depressed, are we likely to do more or fewer pleasant activities?**
      (Answer: We're likely to do fewer pleasant activities and be less active.)
   c. **If we do fewer pleasant activities, are we likely to feel better or worse?**
      (Answer: We will generally feel worse.)
   d. **If we do more pleasant activities, are we likely to feel better or worse?**
      (Answer: We will feel better.)

Now let's look at the second question.

2. What patterns are there?

You might notice patterns in the data on this type of chart. For example, you might tend to feel worse on Mondays when you have to go back to school. Or you might feel worse on weekends when you don't have a regular routine.

    a. **Do you notice any patterns in Susan's chart?**
       (Answer: Yes.)

    b. **What was the lowest number of daily pleasant activities for Susan, and on which day did this occur?**
       (Answer: Two pleasant activities, on Day 14.)

    c. **What do you notice about her mood on that day?**
       (Answer: Susan's mood level was very low, and it was the lowest of all one day before that.)

IV. BASELINE STUDY OF PLEASANT ACTIVITIES (35 min.)

Objectives

1. To help students identify the pleasant activities that have the most influence on mood.
2. To have each student select twenty activities that he or she would like to study and eventually increase.

Important Pleasant Activities

There are some pleasant activities that have been found to be especially important for depression. These are called *MOOD-RELATED ACTIVITIES*. There are two types of mood-related activities that are particularly effective in reducing depression.

1. PLEASANT SOCIAL ACTIVITIES. **Time spent with other people (friends, family) that are positive, pleasurable, and fun.**

2. SUCCESS ACTIVITIES. **Experiences that make us feel skillful or competent (the way we feel when we have done a good job on something).**

| WORKBOOK |

Ask students to answer question #4 on page 2.3.

<u>Leader</u>: Review the correct answers to question #4 as a group when everyone has finished.

Now I want you to answer question #5 at the bottom of the page. Think about yourself for a moment. Which category of activities would make you feel happiest if you did more of it—*social* activities or *success* activities? Write your answer in the space provided.

Follow Up on Simple Baseline Count

Let's look at your baseline count of contributions in class at the top of page 2.2. Does the number surprise you?

<u>Leader</u>: Count the number of slash marks on the blackboard out loud. Comment on how many questions you asked. Point out that counting this action made you more aware of doing it and helped you notice other factors associated with it, such as asking questions when it was quieter in the group, etc.

Did you find that you made more contributions in class because you were paying more attention by keeping a baseline of it? Did you notice any reasons for contributing or not contributing?

This is how we do a baseline. Now you're going to decide which pleasant activities to count.

Selecting Pleasant Activities

Several weeks ago during the intake interview, we asked you to look at a list of pleasant activities and indicate how much you would enjoy each activity and how often you did it. Today, we will be using information from those lists to help us do a baseline like Susan's. The baseline information will be used later to develop a plan for increasing your level of pleasant activities.

| WORKBOOK | Ask students to turn to pages 2.4 and 2.5. |

The Baseline of Pleasant Activities form on page 2.4 will be used to record pleasant activities during the next two weeks.

Leader: Give each student a printout of his or her responses on the Pleasant Events Schedule—Adolescent Version, filled out earlier. If the scored results for the Pleasant Events Schedule are not available for any student, have that student review the items on a blank PES and select those items that seem to meet the criteria on page 2.5 (that is, activities that are frequent, fun, low cost, not objectionable to parents or teachers, observable, and under the control of the student). Emphasize the social activities, since these are the most important for lifting depression.

Follow the directions on page 2.5 and select some pleasant activities for baselining.

Leader: Set a *10-minute* time limit for the students to read the directions and fill out the tracking form. Go around the room as they work and help the slower students.

Instructions for Baselining Pleasant Activities

Part of your assignment for this session is to do a baseline count of how many days these pleasant activities occur. This is how you do it. Simply make a checkmark in the box for the day if the activity occurs at all. For example, if you listen to the radio once or twice in one day, you would simply make one checkmark in the box by that activity for that day. *At the end of each day*, just sit down and think through the day, checking each of the pleasant activities you engaged in.

At the same time, you should also fill out your Mood Diary (page 1.1). If you notice any *patterns* or *reasons* for doing more or fewer activities, write some notes about this in the margin of the diary.

In doing self-observing, it's helpful to maintain an *OBJECTIVE ATTITUDE*. That is, make an effort to record the data accurately. The goal is for you to learn something about yourself. You are not trying to prove anything to anybody, and *you are not attempting to change at this point*. You are just studying your own behavior to see how your activity level and your mood are related.

V. HOMEWORK ASSIGNMENT (10 min.)

| WORKBOOK |

Ask students to turn to the homework assignment on page 2.6.

1. Try to meet the second goal on your Session Goal Record (page 1.2), which is to start two conversations. The person can be someone you know, but try to do it at least once with someone who is normally shy or reluctant to talk with other people. If you reach your goal, mark the box on the Session Goal Record.

2. Take baseline data on your pleasant activities each day, using the form on page 2.4.

3. Fill out your Mood Diary on page 1.1 every day as before.

4. Continue to practice your "friendly skill" (goal #1 on page 1.2), but you don't have to count it this week.

Are there any questions?

Success Activity

Let's do our homework for today.

1. Fill out your Mood Diary for today (page 1.1).

2. Then, fill out the Baseline of Pleasant Activities form on page 2.4 for today. Look at the first activity on your list. Did you do that activity today? If you did, put a checkmark for Day 1 beside that activity. Now look at the next activity. Put a checkmark in the box if you did it today. Continue doing this all the way through your list.

3. Before you leave, start a conversation and practice your friendly skill. Now, you're already halfway to achieving your weekly goal! If you start just one more conversation, you will have met your goal for Session 2.

Preview the Next Session

1. Next session, we'll learn a relaxation technique.

2. **Our baseline study of pleasant activities will continue for two weeks. During the next two sessions, we'll develop a plan for increasing pleasant activities in order to change our moods.**

VI. QUIZ (5 min.)

| WORKBOOK | Ask students to take the quiz on self-observation and change on page 2.7. |

Leader: After everyone has finished, read the answers out loud and have each student correct his or her own quiz.

SESSION 2 QUIZ
Self-Observation and Change

---

1. Put a checkmark next to the situations that would be appropriate times to start a conversation.

    _____ The person is eating as fast as he can.

    _____ The person is walking quickly and doesn't look right or left.

    _✓_ The person smiles at you when you sit down next to him or her.

    _✓_ The person offers you a piece of candy or gum.

    _____ The person looks bored.

2. Put a checkmark next to the questions that would be good for starting a conversation.

    _✓_ Did you hear about [something interesting that happened]?

    _____ What time is it?

    _✓_ What are you going to do when you graduate?

3. Some pairs of activities are listed below. For each pair, put a checkmark next to the activity that would be most effective in lifting depression.

    a. _____ Listening to the radio.
        _✓_ Having friends come over to visit.

    b. _✓_ Meeting someone new that you're attracted to.
        _____ Going horseback riding.

    c. _✓_ Doing a good job at something.
        _____ Throwing a frisbee around.

    d. _✓_ Getting an "A" on a test.
        _____ Watching your favorite TV show.

4. Name the two kinds of information that can be gained from a baseline study of pleasant activities.

    a. Information about how mood and activities are related.

    b. What patterns are there?

SESSION 3
Reducing Tension

Materials needed for this session:
1. Extra workbooks.
2. Extra pens and pencils.
3. Refreshments for the break.
4. Finger thermometers, masking tape.
5. Relaxation audiotapes.

BLACKBOARD

AGENDA
- I. HOMEWORK REVIEW (15 min.)
- II. MEETING NEW PEOPLE (35 min.)
  Break (10 min.)
- III. TENSION (10 min.)
- IV. JACOBSEN RELAXATION TECHNIQUE (25 min.)
- V. QUESTIONS AND ANSWERS (10 min.)
- VI. HOMEWORK ASSIGNMENT (10 min.)
- VII. QUIZ (5 min.)

RULE: Meeting people is a skill you can learn.

I.   HOMEWORK REVIEW (15 min.)

Let's quickly review what we have learned about controlling our moods. This is an oral quiz. I'm going to ask some questions—if you think you know the answer, please raise your hand.

Oral Review/Quiz

1. **What are the three parts of your personality that we talked about in Session 1?**
   (Answer: Actions, thoughts, and feelings.)

2. **How can we use the other two parts to change how we feel?**
   (Answer: We can control our actions and thoughts.)

3. **How do we measure our feelings?**
   (Answer: By filling out the Mood Diary on page 1.1).

4. **What are the four things we can do to be a friendly person?**
   (Answer: Make eye contact, smile, tell about yourself, and say positive things about the other person.)

5. **What are the two types of mood-related activities that are particularly important for reducing depression?**
   (Answer: Pleasant social activities and success activities.)

Review Student Progress/Record Forms

A. **Session Goal (page 1.2)**

   1. **Were you able to meet your goal from the last session, which was to start two conversations?**
   2. **Did you notice situations that would have been good opportunities to start a conversation? Describe some of them.**

<u>Leader</u>: Praise students for noticing situations even if they didn't take advantage of them.

3.   **Did you start a conversation in those situations or did you let the opportunity go by? How did you start the conversation, or why didn't you try?**

Leader: Praise efforts of both kinds.

B.   **Baseline of Pleasant Activities (page 2.4)**

1.   **Did you record your pleasant activities daily? It's important to be accurate when you are collecting this baseline data because you will use it to change the way you feel. The sooner you write down the information, the more accurate it will be.**

Leader: Reward or praise those who recorded their pleasant activities on a daily basis. Hold up several examples of baseline forms that are correctly filled out. Give specific praise for good observing and record-keeping skills. If some students forgot to write down their ratings, have them make retroactive ratings for the past two to four days. (Emphasize, however, that the most accurate ratings are those recorded on a daily basis.)

2.   **Are you noticing things that cause you to do more or fewer pleasant activities? Watch for causes, and write notes about them in your Mood Diary.**

Leader: Ask students to offer examples of some possible causes so they can help each other broaden their ideas of what to look for.

C.   **Mood Monitoring (page 1.1)**

1.   **If you forgot to write down a mood rating, try to recall how you felt, and fill in the number. Remember though, the most accurate ratings are those made on a daily basis.**
2.   **Can you remember some of the events and circumstances that contributed to your high and low mood ratings? Why do you think you felt that way?**
3.   **Have you noticed any improvement in your mood already?**

Leader: Emphasize the importance of daily record keeping. Strongly reinforce those who have been doing it faithfully. Offer some strategies to help those who have been less successful.

D. Other Skills

1. **Did you continue to practice your friendly skill?**
2. **Are you feeling more comfortable in social situations?**

Demonstration Exercise

<u>Leader</u>: Ask teenagers to present new ideas for conversation-starter questions based on any new things they have noticed about people in the course. The time limit for this brief exercise is *5 minutes.*

If we start a conversation we feel in control of the social situation. Feeling in control helps us feel better. It's important to take advantage of opportunities to control our lives.

II. MEETING NEW PEOPLE (35 min.)

Objectives
1. To help students learn how to make a good first impression when they are introduced to a stranger.
2. To show students how to use the same approach when making a self-introduction.

Today, we'll learn another important way to gain control in social situations. We're going to practice the skills that are needed for meeting new people. Meeting new people can make us tense and uncomfortable because we don't know what to expect. The rule for this session is that meeting people is a skill you can learn.

Guidelines for Being Introduced

When you are introduced to someone, you need to remember to do these four things:

BLACKBOARD

> 1. Make eye contact.
> 2. Smile.
> 3. Say a greeting.
> 4. Use the person's name.

If you do these things, the other person will have a good first impression of you, and he or she will be more inclined to like you. *FIRST IMPRESSIONS* are important in establishing relationships. First impressions are remembered for a long time.

Demonstration Exercise

Leader: This is a role-playing exercise, so you will need to ask for a volunteer. The time limit for this exercise is *5 minutes.*

Tell me which person makes a better first impression. Here is Joe (or Beth).

Leader: Have the student introduce you to an imaginary person. Model Joe (or Beth) as a person who looks shyly at his feet when he is introduced and doesn't say anything.

Now, here is Fred (or Sharon).

Leader: Repeat the role-playing exercise, but this time model the four introduction skills that are written on the blackboard.

Which approach makes a better impression?

Choosing a Greeting

Sometimes we don't say anything when we meet people because we're not sure what to say, and the other person seems to do enough talking to fill in the gaps. When you are meeting someone, it's better if each person spends about the same amount of time talking. You will find that it's easier to get a conversation started with someone you don't know if you think of something to say *AHEAD OF TIME*. We're going to plan our greetings now. If you already have a favorite greeting, you might want to think of something better or choose another greeting to alternate with the one you are using now.

```
┌─────────────────┐
│  WORKBOOK       │    Ask students to turn to page 3.1.
└─────────────────┘
```

Look at the menu of greetings near the top of the page. These are some of the greetings that people often use. You can choose one of these or create your own greeting or combination of greetings.

Group Activity

<u>Leader</u>: Have students get together in pairs, or in groups of three. The time limit for this exercise is *5 minutes*.

Discuss these greetings and decide which ones you like, or think of some new ones. Eventually, you need to decide which one you like best and write it in your workbook. You have *5 minutes* to do this.

Some Additional Points

We have been practicing friendly skills, which include making eye contact and smiling. So you are good at this already.

It makes the other person feel noticed if you *REMEMBER HIS OR HER NAME*. Sometimes it's hard to remember people's names, especially if you meet a bunch of new people. We're going to practice saying the person's name at least once at the beginning of the conversation. If you say it once, you will have a better chance of remembering the name so you can use it a second time.

A good way to be sure you use the other person's name at least once is to use it in your greeting. Instead of just saying, "Nice to meet you," you can say, "Nice to meet you, Alice."

SHAKING HANDS is part of the standard adult greeting in our culture; teenagers can do it too, especially when they meet older people. Because shaking hands makes it very apparent that you have noticed the other person, it's a good way to start a conversation with someone you have just met.

We're going to have you practice greetings, including shaking hands.

<u>Leader</u>: Model using all four introduction skills, with a handshake and without.

Demonstration Exercise

Leader: Time limit: *5 minutes*.

I need two people to volunteer for this role-playing exercise. I will introduce you to each other, and you will practice all four of the things needed to make a good first impression.

Leader: After the role play, give each participant specific praise such as "nice smile," "warm-sounding voice," "firm handshake." Avoid criticism. Be sure each of the participants is introduced at least once.

Now I want you to pretend that you're being introduced to an adult. You will need to shake hands this time.

Leader: Ask for additional volunteers, and introduce them in new combinations.

Introducing Yourself to a Stranger

When you introduce yourself to a stranger, you do all of these things and add one more thing—*YOU TELL THE PERSON YOUR NAME*. Customarily, you don't even have to say a whole sentence. You can just greet him or her and say your name, like this.

Leader: Model how this is done by introducing yourself to one of the students.

Group Activity

Time limit: *5 minutes*.

Practice introducing yourself to the person next to you. Pretend you don't know the person. Remember to listen for the person's name. If the person doesn't mention his or her name, you should ask what it is.

Leader: Give specific praise again. Ask a student who is good at introductions to model this for the class.

Break (10 min.)

Let's take a *10-minute* break. Practice your conversation skills during the break by introducing yourself to someone you don't know very well in the group. Also practice starting conversations.

III. TENSION (10 min.)

Objective
1. To help each student evaluate whether tension is a possible problem for him or her.

Tension often gets in the way of doing the things that are necessary to overcome your depression. Situations like meeting new people or starting a conversation can often make you tense, and this tension can make you feel unhappy and nervous. One way to reduce tension in these situations is to practice using social skills such as those presented earlier. There are also some techniques for relaxing that can help. Today we're going to learn a *RELAXATION TECHNIQUE* to help reduce your tension.

To see if the relaxation technique helps, you will need to measure your temperature before we start. What is "measuring the temperature before we start" an example of?
(Answer: Taking a baseline.)

Leader: Before proceeding, have each adolescent tape a finger thermometer to his or her hand. Make sure the bulb of the thermometer is lightly but securely fastened to the pad of the index finger of the hand the teenager doesn't write with. If it is taped too tightly, the circulation will be restricted, and the thermometer will not work properly. The thermometer must be attached for at least *5 minutes* to obtain an accurate reading.

> WORKBOOK   Ask students to turn to page 3.2.

The questions on this page will help you find out if tension is a problem for you. Answer questions #1 through #9 as I read them out loud.

Leader: Reading the questions out loud will circumvent any possible reading problems.

All of these are indicators of tension. If you marked "often" on any of the questions, then learning to relax could be helpful for you.

Leader: Have students read their "before" finger temperature and *RECORD* it on page 3.2. Make a reliability check on each teenager's temperature. Students should also *CIRCLE THE APPROPRIATE NUMBER* at the top of page 3.2 to indicate how relaxed or tense they feel.

IV. THE JACOBSEN RELAXATION TECHNIQUE (25 min.)

Objectives
1. To demonstrate how to use the Jacobsen Relaxation Technique.
2. To help each student identify a situation in his or her life in which prior relaxation would have been most helpful.

Introduce the Jacobsen Relaxation Technique

The relaxation procedures we're going to learn are not hypnosis; they are skills that require conscious work and practice.

The Jacobsen Relaxation Technique is useful for:
1. **Demonstrating how deep relaxation feels (that is, exactly how relaxed you *can* get.)**
2. **Helping you to recognize when you are tense so you can remind yourself to relax.**
3. **Keeping your general tension level down by practicing on a daily basis (even if you aren't tense at the time).**

Leader: Use the relaxation audiotape available from the publisher as a model for your voice. It is important for your voice to reflect the appropriate phase of the tension-release cycle. You should speak somewhat louder and faster during the tension phase and gradually progress to a slower, almost hypnotic-like, soft monotone during the relaxation phase. Tense and relax your own muscles as you go through the exercise to help you control your voice.

As you observe the students tensing and relaxing, give specific correction, feedback, and praise for appropriate tensing and relaxing, while maintaining the appropriate level of voice tension.

One or more students in the group may giggle or be disruptive in other ways during relaxation practice. If this is expected (based on experiences with previous exercises), use some or all of the following techniques to minimize the impact of disruptive behavior: (a) have all of the students turn their chairs around so they are facing away from the table; this minimizes the giggling that occurs when they open their eyes and see everyone else reclined in their chairs; (b) talk with the disruptive student before the relaxation session and emphasize that his or her cooperation is important; (c) place the disruptive student in a chair next to you so you can place your hand on his or her arm if necessary; (d) as a last resort, have the disruptive student practice the relaxation technique in a chair just outside the door.

Demonstration Exercise

1. ***TENSE YOUR ARMS AND HANDS.* Tighten your fists. Don't clench your teeth—just focus on your arms and hands. Make the muscles in your arms as tight as you can.**

Leader: Have students tense for *5-7 seconds.*

Now *RELAX* your arms and hands. Imagine all the energy going out of your arms through your fingertips. Your arms are as relaxed as spaghetti noodles. You couldn't lift a feather.

2. ***TENSE YOUR FACE AND HEAD.* Lift your eyebrows, squint your eyes, clench your teeth. Make every muscle in your head as tight as you possibly can.**

Leader: Have students tense for *5-7 seconds.*

Now *RELAX* your face and head. Let your jaw relax, your eyelids close, and your eyebrows relax. Now all of the energy is leaving your face.

3. ***TENSE YOUR SHOULDERS AND BACK, CHEST, AND STOMACH.* Take a deep breath and hold it. Make your shoulders and back as tight as you can. Pull your stomach muscles up tight. Don't tighten your arms, just your chest and main body. Hold it. Keep it tight, tight, tight.**

<u>Leader</u>: Have students tense for *5-7 seconds*.

> **Now *RELAX*. Breathe out, and let yourself breathe normally. Relax all of those muscles. Notice your deep, rhythmic breathing and the pleasant sensations it produces.**

> 4. *TENSE YOUR LEGS*. **Tense your thighs. Lift your legs slightly off the ground. Press your knees together. Tighten your calves. Press your toes against the floor. Tighten your feet. Turn them up and point them toward your head.**

<u>Leader</u>: Have students tense for only *3-5 seconds* this time, since cramps develop easily in this area.

> **Now *RELAX*. Let all of the tension in your body go out through the tips of your toes. Every last drop of energy is gone from your body. You are totally relaxed. Imagine yourself on a warm beach with the sun shining on your totally relaxed body. You don't have a care in the world.**

<u>Leader</u>: Wait *3-5 minutes*, with occasional instructions to keep breathing regularly and to relax tight muscles.

> *SLOWLY OPEN YOUR EYES*. **Move your arms and legs, wiggle your fingers and toes. Slowly bring your body back to normal. As soon as you are ready, read the temperature on your finger thermometer.**

> *RECORD* **your "after" temperature on page 3.2. Also *CIRCLE A NUMBER* to indicate how relaxed you feel after doing the relaxation exercise. How did you feel during the exercise?**

<u>Leader</u>: Trouble-shoot any problems. Common problems include muscle pains and intrusive thoughts. Describe some alternate ways to tense muscles. Intrusive thoughts are normal, but they can be minimized by concentrating on relaxation.

> **Did relaxation help you? Did your "before" and "after" finger temperature and relaxation ratings change?**

<u>Leader</u>: Briefly explain why relaxation causes an increase in finger temperature, i.e., blood vessels expand which makes extremities warmer.

111

Pinpointing Situations in Which Prior Relaxation Would Be Helpful

| WORKBOOK | Ask students to turn to page 3.3. |

On page 3.3, check the situations that make you feel particularly uncomfortable and tense. If you can think of any other situations, add them to the list in the spaces provided.

| WORKBOOK | Ask students to turn to page 1.2. |

For Session 3 on your Session Goal Record, write . . .

BLACKBOARD

Jacobsen technique 3 times

I'm going to give each of you an audiotape to help you do the relaxation practice.

Leader: Give the relaxation audiotapes to students (these are available from the publisher).

Do this practice before tense situations, like the ones you checked in your workbook on page 3.3.

V. QUESTIONS AND ANSWERS (10 min.)

By this time, you have had a chance to see what this group is like. We've met a few times, you have started to get to know each other, and you have done several exercises together.

Before we talk about the homework assignment, I want to give you a chance to ask questions or express opinions about the course itself and the ideas we have discussed so far. You can ask about anything that's related to the course. I may not be able to answer all of your questions, but I'm willing to try.

<u>Leader</u>: Allow students to discuss, ask questions, and comment about each other or about you. Answer their questions as well as you can. If you aren't able to answer some of the questions, ask your supervisor, and pass the information along to the students during the next session. Limit the time you spend doing this to *10 minutes*.

VI. HOMEWORK ASSIGNMENT (10 min.)

| WORKBOOK | Ask students to turn to the homework assignment on page 3.4.

1. Practice your session goal, which is to do the Jacobsen Relaxation Technique at least three times between now and the next session.

2. Continue to record pleasant activities every day using the form on page 2.4. Look for things that cause you to do more or fewer pleasant activities.

3. Fill out your Mood Diary every day (page 1.1).

4. Continue to practice your friendly skills, including starting conversations with people. If you have the opportunity to meet someone new, practice the introductions we learned today.

Are there any questions?

Success Activity

Let's do our homework for today.

1. We practiced the Jacobsen Relaxation Technique today, so you're already one-third of the way to meeting your session goal. Now you only have to practice two more times. If possible, try to practice more than twice. It makes us feel good to go beyond our goals.

2. Check the pleasant activities you did today on your Pleasant Activities Baseline form on page 2.4.

3. Fill out your Mood Diary for today (page 1.1).

4. Practice introducing yourself to someone right now.

Leader: Allow only *2 minutes* for this practice.

Preview the Next Session

Next session, we'll look closely at your baseline of pleasant activities and make a plan for change. So try to keep good records of your baseline!

VII.   QUIZ (5 min.)

| WORKBOOK |

Ask students to take the quiz on reducing tension on page 3.5.

Leader: After everyone has finished, read the answers out loud and have each student correct his or her own quiz.

SESSION 3 QUIZ
Reducing Tension

1. What are the four things we should remember to do when we meet new people?

   a. _Make eye contact_

   b. _Smile_

   c. _Say a greeting_

   d. _Use the person's name_

2. What can interfere with our ability to enjoy pleasant activities and social interactions?

   Tension, fear, anxiety

3. Is tension a problem for you?　　　　　　　⌐Optional⌐

   　　　　　　　　　　　　　　　　Yes　　　No

   How do you know? _(List physical symptoms from workbook page 3.2, or other signs of anxiety)_

4. Is it possible for people to control tension?　　(Yes)　　No

   How? _By practicing relaxation techniques_

5. Describe a situation in which it would be helpful for you to do the Jacobsen Relaxation Technique ahead of time.

   (e.g., some scheduled event such as a test)

6. In Session 1, we discussed the idea that our personality is a three-part system. What are the three parts? (Hint: Remember the triangle?)

   Feelings, thoughts, behavior

SESSION 4
Learning How to Change

Materials needed for this session:
1. Extra workbooks.
2. Refreshments for the break.
3. Calculators (students can share).
4. Colored pencils or pens (preferably the same two colors for each student).
5. Extra copies of the graph on page 4.1.

BLACKBOARD

AGENDA

 I. HOMEWORK REVIEW (15 min.)

 II. LOOKING AT THE BASELINE INFORMATION (30 min.)

  Break (10 min.)

 III. SETTING GOALS FOR PLEASANT ACTIVITIES (35 min.)

 IV. CONTRACTING (15 min.)

 V. HOMEWORK ASSIGNMENT (10 min.)

 VI. QUIZ (5 min.)

RULE: *You* can learn how to change the way you are.

I.   HOMEWORK REVIEW   (15 min.)

Let's begin this session with a quick review of important points from previous sessions. I'm going to ask some questions—please raise your hand if you think you know the answer.

Oral Review/Quiz

1. **What are four things we should remember to do when we are introduced to people?**
   (Answer: Make eye contact, smile, greet them, use the person's name.)

2. **What are the four friendly skills?**
   (Answer: Smile, make eye contact, tell about yourself, say positive things about the other person.)

3. **What two types of activities are associated with a better mood?**
   (Answer: Pleasant social activities and success activities.)

4. **What can interfere with our ability to enjoy pleasant activities and spend time with other people?**
   (Answer: Tension, anxiety, and having to do other things that interfere.)

5. **What can we do about tension?**
   (Answer: Learn social skills, and practice relaxation techniques like the Jacobsen technique.)

Review Student Progress/Record Forms

A. Session Goal (page 1.2)

1. **Did you practice the Jacobsen Relaxation Technique at least once?** [If necessary, problem solve with students to help them come up with better strategies for managing time, etc.]
2. **Did you schedule practice sessions before high tension situations?**
3. **Do you think the practice helped?**

Group Activity

<u>Leader</u>: Guide students through a brief, *5-minute* relaxation exercise (use the procedures in Session 3 of this manual).

B. Baseline of Pleasant Activities (page 2.4)

1. **Have you been checking your pleasant activities every day?**

C. Mood Monitoring (page 1.1)

1. **Did you have any problems making ratings?**

<u>Leader</u>: If students forgot to make ratings, have them make retroactive ratings for the past two to four days. Emphasize, however, that the most accurate ratings are those made on a daily basis.

2. **Look at the last two weeks in your Mood Diary. Do you see any improvement in your mood?**

D. Social Skills

1. **Did you have any opportunities to practice the introduction skills we learned last session?**
2. **Let's practice right now by introducing yourself to the person sitting next to you.**

<u>Leader</u>: Limit introductions to *1 or 2 minutes* each.

II. LOOKING AT THE BASELINE INFORMATION (30 min.)

Objectives
1. To demonstrate how to chart baseline data for pleasant activities and mood.
2. To help students learn how to analyze baseline data.

Our purpose in this course is to improve the way we feel. Today, we're going to discuss how we can use information from self-observation to decide which changes will help the most, and then we'll consider some effective ways to follow through and make those changes.

The rule for this session is that *YOU* can learn how to change the way you are. *LEARNING TO CHANGE IS DIFFERENT THAN WILLPOWER.* Learning to change is a *SKILL* you can improve with practice. It's not a question of willpower.

There are three critical ingredients for learning to change:
1. *RECOGNIZING THAT YOU CAN LEARN HOW TO CHANGE.* We have already discussed this.
2. *BELIEVING THAT YOU CAN CHANGE.* It's important to have confidence in your ability to change. Do you believe that you can change?
3. *DEVELOPING A PLAN FOR CHANGE.* This is what we're going to do today.

The first step in developing a plan for change is to observe yourself. We have been doing that for one week. The next step is to chart the self-observation information so we can see what's happening.

Charting the Information

| WORKBOOK | Ask students to look at the Baseline of Pleasant Activities form on page 2.4.

1. Put a checkmark by the pleasant activities you did today if you haven't done this already.

2. Now we're going to add up the checkmarks by going down each column. Write the totals for each column at the bottom of the page on the line that says "Totals for Each Day."

Leader: Model how to do this by holding up a copy of page 2.4 that has been filled out with the totals computed.

| WORKBOOK | Ask students to turn to the graph on page 4.1. Have some extra copies available in case students make mistakes.

3. First, we're going to chart our pleasant activities. Look at the numbers on the side of the chart where it says "Daily Total of Pleasant Activities."

Leader: Draw a large scale model of the chart on the blackboard. Ask students to respond as a group to the following questions. When a wrong answer is given, state the correct answer without naming the student who made the error, and then repeat the question.

4. **How many activities does this point represent?**

Leader: (Point to various places on the scale; for example, 6 activities, etc.).

5. **See this line between 10 and 12. [Point.] How many activities does this line represent?**

6. **Where would you put the point to indicate 7 activities for a given day? Where would it be for 17 activities?**

Leader: Continue asking questions using different values until all students answer correctly on four values in a row.

7. **Use a black pen or pencil to make points on the chart representing the total number of pleasant activities you did each day. *DON'T DRAW THE CONNECTING LINES YET.***

Leader: Make up seven data points to use as an example, and write the numbers on the blackboard. Involve the students in deciding where to mark the data points on the chart that you have already drawn on the blackboard. Draw lines connecting the points on the chart.

8. **Now I'm going to check the data points that each of you has marked on your chart. Then I'll give you the go-ahead to draw lines connecting the points.**

Leader: Check the accuracy of each student's data points, then give the go-ahead to draw the connecting lines.

| WORKBOOK | Ask students to turn to the Mood Diary on page 1.1.

9. **We started counting pleasant activities during Session 2, so you should have six or seven days of pleasant activities data. We began recording mood ratings during Session 1, which was several days earlier, so you should have a few more data points for this. You should have nine or ten days of mood rating data.**

For this chart, we want to use the mood ratings that cover the *SAME DAYS* as the pleasant activities ratings. Look for the mood ratings for the *FIRST DAY OF SESSION 2*. This is where you want to start.

10. Look at the chart on page 4.1 again. On one side of the chart it says "Daily Mood Rating." The numbers on this side range from 1 to 7. This is the scale you use to put your mood ratings on the chart.

<u>Leader</u>: Make sure students understand how to use the Daily Mood Rating scale before proceeding. If necessary, use the same line of questioning as the one used to help students understand the pleasant activities scale (for example, "If I wanted to indicate a mood rating of 5 for Day 2, where would I mark the point?").

11. Now you're ready to mark your mood ratings on page 4.1.

12. Use a red pen or pencil (or any different color) to plot the mood rating data points for each day. Be sure to look at the Daily Mood Rating scale when you are marking the points. *DON'T DRAW THE CONNECTING LINES UNTIL I HAVE CHECKED YOUR WORK.*

<u>Leader</u>: Make up seven data points to use as an example, and write the numbers on the side of the blackboard. Involve the students in deciding where to mark the points on the chart you have drawn on the blackboard. Draw the lines connecting the points on the chart.

13. I'm going to check the mood rating points you have marked on your chart, then you can draw the lines connecting the points.

Analyzing the Data

| WORKBOOK |

Ask students to turn to page 4.2.

Answer the questions in Part A. Stop after question #4 and put your pencils down.

<u>Leader</u>: As students work through the questions, walk around the room and offer assistance.

Now you need to decide on a goal. This involves choosing a mood level that you would like to stay above. I'm going to read two examples to illustrate how to choose a *REALISTIC GOAL*.

EXAMPLE 1. **Fred decides he wants to stay at or above a mood level of 4. This is a good goal for Fred because when his mood falls below 4, he feels terrible.**

EXAMPLE 2. **Sally decides she wants to stay at or above a mood level of 7 because she wants to feel great all the time. This is not a realistic goal, however, because it's impossible to feel great all the time.**

Leader: Ask students to read question #5 in Part B, on page 4.2. Help them select a goal of 3, 4, or 5. Each student's choice should be a little higher than his or her lowest mood level. Encourage students to discuss the reasons for their choices. Use the following questions to guide the discussion.

Why did you choose this number as your goal? Is it just a little higher than your lowest mood level? If not, you should consider choosing another goal. We want you to be successful in meeting your goal, so it's important to be realistic. You can always raise your goal to a higher mood level later on.

Draw a colored line on your chart at the mood level you have selected as your goal, like this.

Leader: Demonstrate this for students by choosing a mood level and drawing a corresponding line on the blackboard chart.

Break (10 min.)

Let's take a *10-minute* break.

III. SETTING GOALS FOR PLEASANT ACTIVITIES (35 min.)

Objectives
1. To review the characteristics of good goals.
2. To help each student identify the pleasant activities that would have the most impact on his or her mood if they were increased.
3. To assist students in developing strategies for increasing the number of pleasant activities.

Setting Appropriate Goals

Goals Must Be Specific

BLACKBOARD

Poor Goals:
I want to do more pleasant activities.
I want to succeed.

The reason these are examples of poor goals is that they are *NOT SPECIFIC ENOUGH*. This means it would be very difficult to know whether you have actually reached the goal. The following are some examples of good goals.

BLACKBOARD

Good Goals:
I want to call my best friend once every day.
I want to join a horse club.

Goals Must Be Realistic

BLACKBOARD

Poor Goals:
I want to increase my daily average of pleasant activities from 2 per day to 10 per day.
I want to get straight A's *every* semester.

Good goals lead to improvement through *SMALL, REALISTIC STEPS*.

Leader: Convert the examples of poor goals to good goals (for example, increase the level of pleasant activities from 2 per day to 4 per day). Solicit suggestions from students about how to change the examples, and guide the process by providing feedback and explanations.

Good goals are a *SMALL IMPROVEMENT* over your baseline level.

┌─────────────┐
│ WORKBOOK │   Ask students to turn to page 4.3.
└─────────────┘

Write the two characteristics of good goals at the top of page 4.3.

Leader: Correct the students' answers immediately.

The example at the top of page 4.3 is about the data Mary collected on pleasant activities and mood ratings. Let's read the example together.

Leader: Read the example about Mary out loud as the students follow along in the workbook.

What would be good pleasant activities goals for Mary?
(Answer: A minimum of 3 pleasant activities per day, and maintaining her average of 5 would be good goals for Mary.)

Now decide what would be good pleasant activities goals for you, and write them at the bottom of page 4.3. You may find it useful to review pages 4.1 and 4.2. Think about the goal you set for mood level.

┌─────────────┐
│ WORKBOOK │   Ask students to turn to the Session Goal Record on page 1.2.
└─────────────┘

The goal for Session 4 is to do the number of pleasant activities you have indicated at the bottom of page 4.3. Write "Do [your specific number] of pleasant activities each day" on the line for Session 4.

Identifying "High Impact" Activities

There are certain activities that make the most difference in your mood if you increase them. Some activities are just more "powerful" than other, more ordinary activities. What are some "high impact" or "powerful" activities for each of you?

Leader: Write the students' answers on the blackboard.

You should try to focus on increasing these activities.

Looking for Causes

Sometimes we find that our levels of pleasant activities are controlled by other things. For example, we might not do many pleasant activities on Mondays because we have to get back to the school routine and we feel down, or we might not do social activities unless someone invites us.

| WORKBOOK | Ask students to read questions #1 and #2 on page 4.4. |

Team Activity

Leader: Have students form teams by pairing up (or have them form groups of three if there is an uneven number of students).

The next step is for you to help your teammate answer questions #1 and #2.

Did you find that there are some events and patterns associated with your level of pleasant activities?

Leader: Use the information offered by students to generate examples for the discussion that follows.

Increasing Pleasant Activities

We want to think of some ways to increase our levels of pleasant activities. The simplest approach would be to try to do pleasant activities more often. But for some of you, it may not be that easy. There might be a *PATTERN* in your life that will make it difficult for you to increase these activities, unless we come up with some ideas for making it easier.

For example, if pleasant *SOCIAL ACTIVITIES* would make you feel happiest, but you never do anything with people except go to classes where you're not supposed to talk, it might be difficult for you to increase those activities. One way to improve the situation would be for you to set a goal to *JOIN A CLUB*. This could be a school club, a church teen group, or some other club that would give you an opportunity to be with other people in a casual situation.

If *SUCCESS ACTIVITIES* would make you feel happiest, but there aren't enough things that you feel you do well, then you might need to *SET A GOAL TO LEARN HOW TO DO SOMETHING BETTER*. This may involve taking lessons, or joining a hobby group.

If you find you don't do a pleasant activity unless it's *SOMEONE ELSE'S IDEA* and he or she invites you, then you might need to begin thinking of pleasant activities and *INVITE OTHERS TO JOIN YOU*.

Leader: Create some additional examples that relate directly to the students' responses to questions #1 and #2.

Ask students to read question #3 on page 4.4.

Think about how you could increase the opportunities available to you for doing pleasant activities. Write your ideas in the space provided after question #3.

Now I want you to work on this with your teammate. Decide which of you will start first, and focus on that person's answers to question #2. Come up with some ways to change each situation so that pleasant activities will happen more often. You will have about *3 minutes* to do this, and then I will signal that it's time to focus on the other person's answers to question #2. OK, let's begin right now.

Leader: Wait *3 minutes*, then give a verbal cue that it is time for the other person to take a turn. The students will probably need some guidance in determining appropriate strategies. Walk around the room while the groups are working and offer assistance.

What are some of the things you decided would help you increase your opportunities for pleasant activities? As you hear good ideas from others that you could use, add them to your list under question #3.

Now I want you to consult with your teammate to decide which idea listed under question #3 would make the most difference for you in terms of increasing pleasant activities. Place a *STAR* by that idea or strategy.

IV. CONTRACTING (15 min.)

Objectives
1. To have each student create a list of rewards that he or she has control over.
2. To help each student develop a personal contract.

It has been demonstrated that you are more likely to meet your goals if you make a written contract with yourself. In this case, the contract is a formal agreement to reward yourself if you accomplish your goals.

Selecting a Reward

Selecting a good reward is an important part of making your contract work. There are certain rules for selecting good rewards:

1. **They should be *SOMETHING YOU REALLY ENJOY*. Don't pick them because you think you *should* enjoy them. For example, going to a party would be a bad reward if you hate parties.**

2. **They should be *UNDER YOUR CONTROL*. The reward should be readily available, not something that someone else has to get for you. For example, driving the car would be a bad reward if you don't have a car.**

3. **They should be *POWERFUL*. The reward should be equal to the effort you put into meeting your goals. For example, going to a movie would be a more powerful reward than chewing gum.**

4. **They should be *IMMEDIATELY AVAILABLE* when you meet your goal. Don't make yourself wait for the reward. For example, listening to your favorite album would be a bad reward if you won't be able to do it until later that day.**

WORKBOOK   Ask students to turn to page 4.5.

Leader: Have students complete the Reward Selection Worksheet. Move on to the next section after everyone has finished.

Writing a Contract

WORKBOOK   Ask students to turn to page 4.6.

Help your teammate write a Pleasant Activities Contract, using all of the information from earlier in today's session.

V. HOMEWORK ASSIGNMENT (10 min.)

WORKBOOK   Ask students to turn to the homework assignment on page 4.7.

1. **Try to meet your goal for Session 4, which is to maintain your pleasant activities at a specific level. Follow the terms of your contract on page 4.6 by keeping track of whether you achieve your goals on a daily and weekly basis; give yourself the reward you have selected if you're successful.**

2. **Continue recording your pleasant activities on page 2.4.**

3. **Fill out your Mood Diary (page 1.1) every day.**

4. **You may want to practice the Jacobsen Relaxation Technique, especially before stressful situations.**

Are there any questions?

Success Activity

Let's do our homework for today.

1. Check the pleasant activities that you did today on page 2.4.

2. If you checked enough activities to meet your daily goal, put a checkmark in the appropriate box on page 4.6, and check the box on your Session Goal Record (page 1.2).

Preview the Next Session

Next session, we'll begin to learn about controlling our thinking. We'll also check to see if you were able to meet your contract goals.

VI. QUIZ (5 min.)

| WORKBOOK | Ask students to take the quiz on learning how to change on page 4.8. |

<u>Leader</u>: After everyone has finished, read the answers out loud and have each student correct his or her own quiz.

SESSION 4 QUIZ
Learning How to Change

1. Put the following steps for developing and implementing a plan for change in the correct sequence (1 = first step, 2 = second step, etc.).

   __3__ Look closely at the baseline information.

   __1__ Select a specific behavior or problem situation to observe.

   __5__ Choose a reward and make a contract with yourself.

   __7__ Reward yourself.

   __4__ Set a realistic goal for improvement.

   __2__ Observe yourself and take a baseline count.

   __6__ Meet your goal.

2. Name two characteristics of good goals.

   a. __Small, realistic__   b. __Specific (concrete)__

3. Mary never goes anywhere unless someone invites her. What would be a good goal for Mary that would help her increase her pleasant activities?

   ___To invite other people to do things___

Continued on the next page

EXTRA CREDIT

4. Come up with a good goal for Carlos and write it below.

    The Situation. Carlos found that his mood and the number of pleasant activities he did were closely related. One day, he did 15 pleasant activities, and the next day his mood rating was 7, its highest point for the two-week period. On another day, he did no pleasant activities at all, and his mood rating was only 2. His mood ratings fell below 5 only eleven times out of the fourteen days; during these periods, his pleasant activities level was often below 2. His average daily number of pleasant activities was 3.

    Good goals for Carlos:
    Average daily number of pleasant activities __4__.
    Minimum level of pleasant activities __3__.

1 pt.
1 pt.

SESSION 5
Changing Your Thinking

Materials needed for this session:
1. Extra workbooks.
2. Refreshments for the break.
3. Colored pens or pencils (preferably the same two colors for each student).
4. Calculators (students can share).
5. A pack of 3" x 5" index cards.

BLACKBOARD

AGENDA
- I. HOMEWORK REVIEW (20 min.)
- II. HOW TO MAKE A PLAN WORK (15 min.)
- III. CONVERSATION SKILLS (15 min.)
  - *Break (10 min.)*
- IV. CONTROLLING YOUR THINKING (45 min.)
- V. HOMEWORK ASSIGNMENT (10 min.)
- VI. QUIZ (5 min.)

RULE: Plan for success.

I. HOMEWORK REVIEW (20 min.)

Let's quickly review some important points from the previous sessions. This is an oral quiz. I'm going to ask some questions—please raise your hand if you think you know the answer.

Oral Review/Quiz

1. **Your personality is a three-part system. What are the parts?**
    (Answer: Actions/behavior, thoughts, and feelings.)

2. **Which two parts are easiest to change?**
    (Answer: Actions/behavior and thoughts.)

3. **Which part have we been learning to change by working on increasing pleasant activities?**
    (Answer: Actions/behavior.)

4. **What are two characteristics of *good* goals?**
    (Answer: They are specific and small/realistic.)

5. **What is a realistic goal?**
    (Answer: A little more than baseline.)

6. **What is baselining?**
    (Answer: Counting how often we do something before we try to change it.)

7. **Why do we do baselining?**
    (Answer: To help us set realistic goals and make a plan for change.)

8. **What can get in the way of our ability to *enjoy* social activities?**
    (Answer: Tension.)

9. **How can we control tension?**
    (Answer: By using relaxation techniques.)

Review Student Progress/Record Forms

A. **Session Goal (page 1.2)**

   1. Were you able to meet your daily goal for pleasant activities on page 4.6? Did you reward yourself?
   2. Will you be able to meet your weekly goal tomorrow? If you are successful, be sure to give yourself the bigger reward.
   3. Do you feel that increasing pleasant activities is helping you change your mood?

B. **Pleasant Activities (page 2.4)**

   1. Did you baseline pleasant activities on a daily basis?

C. **Mood Monitoring (page 1.1)**

   1. Did you remember to fill out your Mood Diary every day?

D. **Graphing Pleasant Activities and Mood Ratings (page 4.1)**

   1. First, total the daily number of pleasant activities on page 2.4.
   2. Mark the data points for pleasant activities on the graph on page 4.1. Connect the points with lines using the same color of pen or pencil as you used last time for pleasant activities.
   3. Mark the mood ratings from page 1.1 on the graph on page 4.1. Connect the points with lines using the same color of pen or pencil as you used last time for mood ratings.
   4. Calculate your average number of pleasant activities and average mood rating since last session.

   If you haven't noticed any changes yet, don't give up—we're just getting started.

E. **Relaxation** (optional)

   1. Did you practice the Jacobsen Relaxation Technique this week?
   2. Are you finding the technique to be useful?

Group Activity

<u>Leader</u>: Guide students through a brief, *5-minute* relaxation exercise using the procedure outlined in Session 3.

F. Social Skills

    1. Did you have an opportunity to practice the introduction skills we learned in Session 3? How did it go?

Demonstration Exercise

<u>Leader</u>: Ask for some volunteers to demonstrate introduction skills. Have them model introducing themselves, introducing others, and being introduced. Time limit: *3 minutes*.

II. HOW TO MAKE A PLAN WORK (15 min.)

Objectives

1. To help each student develop one important strategy for improving his or her success rate on the Pleasant Activities Contract.
2. To have each student evaluate his or her goal for pleasant activities, and make appropriate adjustments.

Group Sharing

What were some things you did that helped you meet your goals? What were some of the problems?

It can be difficult or even scary to *MAKE CHANGES* in our lives. The way things are now—even if they're lousy—is more familiar, "safer," and easier. However, making changes can be helpful and even exciting. We encourage you to view this course as an opportunity and a challenge to make some changes in your life. Experiment with new ways of doing things. We think you will be happy with the results. In the past, you have probably been asked to make changes by someone else—your parents, teachers, etc. In this course, you have the opportunity to *CHOOSE POSITIVE CHANGES FOR YOURSELF*.

Planning for Success

The rule for this session is to *PLAN FOR SUCCESS*.

```
┌─────────────┐
│  WORKBOOK   │      Ask students to turn to page 5.1.
└─────────────┘
```

<u>Leader</u>: As students consider the ideas in the summary that follows, have them put a check mark next to the ones they could use on page 5.1.

Here are some general points to keep in mind:

1. **MAKE A COMMITMENT. When you decide to increase positive activities, you will be making choices, establishing priorities, and rearranging your life a bit. Sometimes it's easier and less frightening to do nothing, even when we aren't happy with conditions as they are right now. Making a commitment to achieve a *SMALL INCREASE* in your pleasant activities is a good first step to gaining control over your life and your mood.**

<u>Leader</u>: The following are some practical suggestions for increasing pleasant activities. Write them on the blackboard, and discuss how each of them could be helpful. Time limit: *4 minutes*.

BLACKBOARD

```
┌──────────────────────────────────────────────────────┐
│   1.  Schedule activities in advance.                 │
│   2.  Don't let yourself back out or make excuses.    │
│   3.  Make a commitment to another person.            │
│   4.  Designate the time and place.                   │
│   5.  Make a "to do" list.                            │
│   6.  Anticipate problems and try to prevent them.    │
└──────────────────────────────────────────────────────┘
```

2. **ACHIEVE A BALANCE. The goal is to achieve a balance between the things you *MUST DO* and the things you *WANT TO DO*.**

Some specific methods for increasing pleasant activities are:

1. *USE STRATEGIES.* Plan time effectively—set aside blocks of time for things you have to do and for pleasant activities. Make a "to do" list. Establish priorities—what do you really need to do?
2. *PLAN AHEAD.* Anticipate problems, and try to prevent them. For example, arrange for transportation ahead of time, make reservations, etc.

Evaluating Goals

Small Group Activity

<u>Leader</u>: Each student who didn't meet his or her goal for pleasant activities needs to develop a clear understanding of *one* important thing he or she could do to increase the likelihood of success. Depending on the number of students and how compatible their personalities are, divide the class into small groups or meet as a large group to work on the tasks below. Time limit: *5 minutes*.

1. Have students review and revise their pleasant activities goals on page 4.6. Students who were able to meet their goals should keep them at the same level or raise them slightly, and those who were not successful should lower their goals.
2. Help students who were not able to meet their goals. Do some brainstorming to come up with strategies that address the factors that got in the way of achieving the goal.

Ask students to answer question #2 on page 5.1.

III. CONVERSATION SKILLS (15 min.)

Objective
1. To practice joining and leaving a conversation group.

We have already discussed how to begin conversations with people. Today we're going to build on what we have learned by practicing *JOINING AND LEAVING CONVERSATION GROUPS*. This is a skill that often comes in handy at social gatherings like weddings and parties. In our culture, it's appropriate to join and leave conversations frequently. The reason people stand up at parties is so they can move around easily from one group to the next. In spite of this, it can sometimes be uncomfortable to join and leave conversation groups.

Joining a Conversation Group

1. **How do you join a group that is talking together?**
    (Answer: Just stand near the group. Often, someone will open up the circle to include you. It isn't necessary to say anything, you can just listen. Sitting far away will not lead to an invitation to join a conversation group.)

Demonstration Exercise

Leader: Ask for three volunteers to form a standing conversation group. Have the group model three approaches to joining a conversation. Participate in the exercise if the students have trouble with some of the examples. Make the role plays very brief. Time limit: *1 minute.*

EXAMPLE 1. Go up to the group and push someone aside.

EXAMPLE 2. Stand far away.

EXAMPLE 3. Stand near the group.

2. **If you are in a conversation group and someone stands behind you, what should you do?**
    (Answer: Open up the circle to include that person.)

3. **How do you know what to say in the conversation?**
    (Answer: When you feel you have something to say, you can join the conversation by asking a question, offering a fact, or telling a story. Your comment should RELATE TO THE TOPIC being discussed. This is also part of being a good listener.)

Leaving a Conversation Group

The conventions for leaving a large group are different than those for leaving a "two-person group" which consists of just you and another person.

1. **How do you leave a large group (consisting of more than just you and another person)?**
    (Answer: This is easy. If the other members of the group are actively involved in a conversation, just say "Excuse me" and leave with a smile or a nod.)

Demonstration Exercise

<u>Leader</u>: Ask for three volunteers to form a standing conversation group. Have them model how to join and leave a large group. Time limit: *3 minutes.*

2. **How do you leave a two-person group that consists of you and one other person?**
   (Answer: This is more difficult. You should say something to end the conversation.)

3. **What are some things you can say to end the conversation?**
   (Answer: "I think I'll get more food or drink," "I'd like to talk to so-and-so over there," or "I'll see you later." You don't have to lie or make big excuses.)

Demonstration Exercise

<u>Leader</u>: Ask a student to help you with this exercise. Briefly model some appropriate and inappropriate ways to initiate and end a conversation with someone. Have students label what was right or wrong with your approach.

Break (10 min.)

Let's take a *10-minute* break. During the break, I want you to practice what we have just learned. Join and leave a conversation group at least once.

IV. CONTROLLING YOUR THINKING (45 min.)

Objectives
1. To help each student identify his or her most frequent negative and positive thoughts.
2. To have each student determine his or her ratio of positive to negative thoughts.
3. To give feedback as the students identify negative thoughts and activating events in cartoon sequences.
4. To have students record daily (for the following week) their worst negative thoughts, the activating events that made them think that way, and the number of times they catch themselves thinking negatively.

We have been working on changing our *ACTIONS* by increasing pleasant activities. Today we're going to start learning how to change our *THINKING*. When people are depressed, they tend to have more negative thoughts and fewer positive thoughts.

1. **What kind of goals would you expect to have for changing your thinking?**
   (Answer: Goals that involve increasing positive thoughts and decreasing negative thoughts.)

2. **Do you believe that you can control your thoughts?**
   *(Answer, if the response is **NO**: We often believe that we can't control our thoughts, but it is possible. We'll be learning some techniques to help us do this during this session and the next one.)*

   *(Answer, if the response is **YES**: Ask students to suggest some specific techniques. Be brief in collecting answers. Confirm that yes, it is possible to control our thinking. We're going to learn several ways to do this.)*

Group Exercise

<u>Leader</u>: Have students *WORRY COVERTLY* (to themselves). After about *20 seconds*, ask them to stop. Now have them *THINK POSITIVE THOUGHTS* for *30 seconds*—ask them to concentrate on pleasant experiences, recall their favorite places, think positive things about themselves, etc. Provide some examples of positive thoughts. Briefly ask them what they experienced. How did their mood change? Point out that they have just controlled their thinking.

Before we can control our thoughts, we must become aware of them. In particular, we need to know which negative thoughts we have most often. Everyone has negative thoughts sometimes, and there are good reasons to have them every now and then. But *NEGATIVE THOUGHTS CAN BECOME A PROBLEM IF THEY OCCUR TOO FREQUENTLY* because they make us feel sad or down. The most effective way to work on negative thoughts is to identify the ones that occur most often.

3. **What is the first step in controlling our thoughts?**
   (Answer: Becoming aware of our thoughts; identifying the negative thoughts we have most often.)

When we become aware of our thoughts, we should notice whether we're thinking more positive thoughts or more negative thoughts. As a general rule of thumb, we should have at least *TWICE AS MANY POSITIVE THOUGHTS AS NEGATIVE THOUGHTS* (although this can vary somewhat from one person to the next).

4. **How many positive thoughts should we have for each negative thought?**
   (Answer: The ratio should be two to one.)

Leader: Ask students to answer questions #3 and #4 on page 5.1.

Identifying Frequent Negative Thoughts

WORKBOOK   Ask students to turn to pages 5.2 and 5.3.

5. **On pages 5.2 and 5.3 there is a list of negative thoughts that tend to occur frequently. Have you had any of these? Check the ones that are familiar to you.**

6. **At the bottom of page 5.3, write down any other negative thoughts that you have had.**

Leader: Give students some time to work. Begin the next exercise when 80% of the students seem to have finished.

To help you identify other negative thoughts, I'm going to describe some situations. I want you to write down any negative or positive thoughts you might have *ABOUT YOURSELF* in each situation. Add these thoughts to the list you have started at the bottom of page 5.3.

   a. **It's Monday, and you find out that some friends of yours went to a movie on Saturday and didn't invite you.**
   b. **Your parents won't let you go to a particular party on Friday night.**
   c. **You have just finished a very hard exam, and your best friend tells you that he or she thought the exam was fairly easy.**
   d. **You see a group of friends having fun together, and you're not with them.**

Now look at your list of negative thoughts.

7. Do you have some of these thoughts much more often than the others? Put a star or an asterisk by the most frequent thoughts. Put two stars or asterisks by the thoughts that are super-frequent.

Identifying Positive Thoughts

WORKBOOK	Ask students to turn to page 5.4.

There is a list of positive thoughts on page 5.4. Read through the list and check the thoughts that you have had during the past month. At the bottom of the page, list some other positive thoughts that you have had.

Comparing the Totals

WORKBOOK	Ask students to turn to page 5.5.

Count the number of positive thoughts you have identified from the list on page 5.4, and write the total on the line provided at the top of page 5.5 (question #5). Then count up the negative thoughts you identified from the list on pages 5.2 and 5.3 and write that total on the next line. Which total is higher—the one for negative thoughts or the one for positive thoughts?

8. You should have twice as many positive thoughts as negative thoughts. Do you?

9. If you want to make a plan for changing your thinking, what should you do first? Here's a hint; what did you do *FIRST* when you worked on changing your level of pleasant activities?
    (Answer: Take baseline data.)

Identifying Activating Events

When you take a baseline on your thinking you will need to notice when you are thinking negatively. When you discover that you are thinking negatively, you will also need to figure out what situation or event caused the negative thinking. We call this the *ACTIVATING EVENT*.

<u>Leader</u>: Write *"Activating Event"* on the blackboard.

We're going to practice identifying activating events by looking at some cartoons.

<u>Leader</u>: Ask students to read question #6 on page 5.5.

Read the Bloom County cartoon and circle the negative thoughts.

1. **What did you circle for the negative thought?**
   (Answer, Opus: "I'm as handsome as I'm gonna get . . . and that's not too handsome.")

Describe the activating event on the line below the cartoon.

2. **What is the activating event?**
   (Answer: Humming a recent Wayne Newton hit.)

WORKBOOK   Ask students to read question #7 on page 5.6.

Read the Garfield cartoon. Circle the negative thought, then describe the activating event on the line below the cartoon.

3. **What did you circle for the negative thought?**
   (Answer, Jon: "I feel like such an unworthy parent.")

4. **What is the activating event?**
   (Answer: Finding Garfield in shock in front of the TV.)

Recording Negative Thoughts

┌─────────────┐
│ WORKBOOK   │ Ask students to turn to page 5.7.
└─────────────┘

The form on page 5.7 is for recording baseline data on negative thoughts. You will use this form to write down your *MOST NEGATIVE THOUGHTS* each day and the *ACTIVATING EVENT* that came before each thought.

Every day for a week, we want you to *RECORD AT LEAST ONE NEGATIVE THOUGHT*—preferably the worst, most depressing thought you had that day. This will be hard to remember from one day to the next, so you'll need to fill out the inventory form every day.

When you realize that you are thinking negatively, also try to identify the activating event that caused you to begin thinking this way. Write down some notes about this as well.

Your goal is to record at least one thought for each day. Another useful piece of information is *HOW MANY TIMES* you caught yourself thinking negatively; write this down in the space provided on the form.

Leader: Emphasize that recording one negative thought each day is critical because the exercises in subsequent sessions are based on this information. The counting part is not as important, but it will also be helpful.

Discuss some ways to take notes on negative thoughts right after they occur. Hand out blank 3" x 5" cards, and suggest using the cards to record thoughts. Help students think of a place in their notebooks or purses to carry the cards. Show some examples of good record keeping.

When you catch yourself thinking negatively, try to think positive thoughts instead. I know this can be very difficult, but give it a try anyway. We'll show you some techniques to make this easier later in the course.

V. HOMEWORK ASSIGNMENT (10 min.)

┌─────────────┐
│ WORKBOOK   │ Ask students to turn to the homework assignment on page 5.8.
└─────────────┘

1. **Your main goal is to increase your pleasant activities so that you consistently meet your daily goal on page 4.6. Turn to page 1.2 and write this as your goal on the line for Session 5.**

2. **Keep recording your pleasant activities on page 2.4.**

Leader: *THIS IS OPTIONAL.* You may want to announce that you have set a goal for the entire group, "If __% of the class meet the daily goal for pleasant activities every day until next session, I will bring _____ for the whole group." Make sure the percentage you use for the goal is a small improvement over the students' performances last week.

3. **Take a baseline of negative thoughts, using page 5.7.**
   a. **Write down your worst negative thought for the day and the event or situation that activated it. Try using the 3" x 5" card to take notes right after the thought occurs, then transfer the notes to page 5.7.**

Leader: Pass out 3" x 5" cards to students.

   b. *OPTIONAL.* **Count the number of times you catch yourself thinking negatively every day and record it on page 5.7.**

4. **Continue to fill out your Mood Diary on page 1.1.**

5. **Practice the Jacobsen Relaxation Technique, especially before stressful situations.**

Are there any questions?

Success Activity

Let's do our homework for today.

1. **Write down at least one of the worst negative thoughts you have had today on page 5.7. Describe the situation or event that made you think this way.**

2. **When you catch yourself thinking negatively this week, what will you do?**
   (Answer: Try to think of some positive thoughts instead.)

3. **Fill out your Mood Diary for today.**

Preview the Next Session

Next session, we'll learn about the power of positive thinking.

VI. QUIZ (5 min.)

WORKBOOK   Ask students to take the quiz on changing your thinking on page 5.9.

Leader: After everyone has finished, read the answers out loud and have each student correct his or her own quiz.

SESSION 5 QUIZ
Changing Your Thinking

1. What is the first step in controlling your thoughts?

   pt.   _Identifying negative thoughts, becoming aware of thoughts_

2. You should have at least **2** positive thoughts for every negative one.

   pt.

3. Circle the negative thought in the following cartoon.

   pt.

CALVIN & HOBBES   **Bill Watterson**

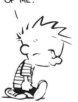
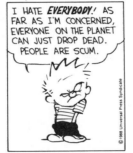
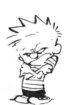
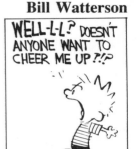

4. What is the Activating Event for the negative thought in the cartoon above?

   1 pt.

   Being in a bad mood.

EXTRA CREDIT

5. Come up with a plan to help Maria increase how often she talks with friends, which is an important pleasant activity for her.

   THE SITUATION. Maria enjoys spending time visiting with her friends and she would like to do this more often. However, Maria feels that she can't go to a friend's house unless she is invited, and she doesn't invite friends to her house because she thinks her house is an ugly mess. What could Maria do to increase how often she visits with her friends?

   pt.

   Invite friends to go out somewhere other than her house; clean up the house, then invite friends, etc.

SESSION 6
The Power of Positive Thinking

Materials needed for this session:
1. Extra workbooks.
2. Extra pens and pencils.
3. Refreshments for the break.
4. Calculators (students can share).
5. Positive statements about each student.
6. *Optional:* Reward for group goal.

BLACKBOARD

AGENDA

  I.   REVIEW HOMEWORK (15 min.)
  II. INCREASING POSITIVE THINKING (25 min.)
  III. IDENTIFYING NEGATIVE THOUGHTS (5 min.)
       Break (10 min.)
  IV. CHANGING NEGATIVE THINKING TO POSITIVE THINKING (50 min.)
  V.   CONTRACT (5 min.)
  VI. HOMEWORK ASSIGNMENT (5 min.)
  VII. QUIZ (5 min.)

RULE: Think positive.

<u>Leader</u>: This is one of the most difficult sessions to complete in two hours. It is important to follow the time suggestions very closely in this session.

I. HOMEWORK REVIEW (15 min.)

Let's begin with a quick review of some of the important points that we have covered so far in this course. I'm going to ask some questions—please raise your hand if you think you know the answer.

Oral Review/Quiz

1. **Identify whether the following are negative thoughts, positive thoughts, or neither:**

THOUGHT	*ANSWER*
"What's the use?"	(-)
"I can't do that!"	(-)
"That's interesting."	(+)
"It's my fault."	(-)
"Fred likes me."	(+)
"I'm a good listener."	(+)

2. **How do you join a conversation group of two or more people at a party?**
   (Answer: Stand near the group and ask questions or make comments related to the topics being discussed.)

3. **How would you leave this conversation group?**
   (Answer: Say "excuse me," smile, and leave.)

4. **How do you start a conversation with someone who is not in a group at a party?**
   (Answer: You go up to him or her and ask a good conversation-starting question.)

5. **How would you end a conversation with that person?**
   (Answer: Say "Excuse me," and/or say what you want to do now, for example, "Well, I'm going to go get something to drink.")

Review Student Progress/Record Forms

<u>Leader</u>: Keep the review moving along. The time limit for each question is *1-2 minutes*.

A. Session Goal (page 1.2)

1. **Did you record your pleasant activities on page 2.4?**
2. **Did you add up the totals for each day?**
3. **How many of you were able to consistently meet your daily goal (page 4.6) for increasing pleasant activities?**

<u>Leader</u>: If you promised a group reward last session and enough students were successful in meeting their daily goals, give the reward. If the reward is something edible, the students can eat it while they chart their mood and pleasant activities data.

B. Graph of Mood and Pleasant Activities (page 4.1)

1. **Plot the data points for pleasant activities (page 2.4) on your graph on page 4.1, and draw the connecting lines with a colored pen or pencil (preferably, use the same color as last time).**
2. **Plot the data points for mood ratings (page 1.1) on the same graph and draw the connecting lines with a colored pen or pencil (preferably, use the same color as last time).**

<u>Leader</u>: Hand out calculators.

3. **Calculate or estimate the average number of pleasant activities you did each day for last week.**
4. **Is your overall average increasing?**
5. **Has there been any improvement in your mood ratings?**
6. **Is your mood staying above your critical level?**
7. **What plan or strategy did you try last week to help you achieve your goals? Did it work?**

C. Social Skills

1. **Did you have an opportunity to practice the skills we learned last week for joining and leaving a conversation? How did it go?**

<u>Leader</u>: Limit responses to an average of *30 seconds* each.

D. Negative Thoughts Baseline (page 5.7)

    1.   **Did you record at least one of your worst negative thoughts each day?**
    2.   **Did you record the activating event for that thought?**

We'll look more closely at your negative thoughts baseline in a few minutes. Before we do that, let's talk about positive thoughts.

II. INCREASING POSITIVE THINKING (25 min.)

Objectives

1.   To help each student come up with at least one positive statement about each person in the room.
2.   To have each student write down the positive statements about him- or herself that are offered by others.

Positive Statements About Each Other

When we think negatively about ourselves, we often think negatively about others. It's good practice to think positively about others and about ourselves. The rule for this session is to think positive.

Group Activity

WORKBOOK	Ask students to turn to page 6.1.

Now I want you to take a few minutes to write one or two *POSITIVE STATEMENTS* about each of the other people in the class. Write these statements down on page 6.1 as you think of them. Make sure you have at least one positive statement for each person. When everyone has finished, each person will read his or her statements out loud. I will demonstrate how to do this by reading the positive statements I have already written about each of you.

<u>Leader</u>: Read the statements you have prepared. Try to focus on good personality traits and habits (e.g., good sense of humor) rather than physical attributes (e.g., attractive). This provides a better model for students.

OK, it's your turn to think of some positive statements—they should be different from mine.

<u>Leader</u>: While the students are working, walk around the room, and help those who are having trouble by whispering some hints.

Recording Positive Statements About Yourself

WORKBOOK

After everyone has finished, ask them to turn to page 6.2.

Now I'm going to have you take turns reading your statements to the rest of the class. As you hear other students say positive things about you, write their comments on page 6.2. Who would like to start?

<u>Leader</u>: If no one volunteers, call on students one at a time. Continue until everyone has had a chance to read his or her statements to the rest of the class. Time limit: *20 minutes.*

III. IDENTIFYING NEGATIVE THOUGHTS (5 min.)

Objectives
1. To distinguish between *PERSONAL* and *NONPERSONAL* negative thoughts.
2. To help each student use baseline information to make a list of the negative personal thoughts that are most troublesome to him or her.

Personal vs. Nonpersonal Negative Thoughts

In learning how to control our thoughts, it's helpful to distinguish between personal and nonpersonal thoughts. Personal thoughts are about yourself. Nonpersonal thoughts are about other people and things. We're going to work on our personal thoughts during this session. In the next session, we'll work on our nonpersonal thoughts that are troublesome.

A personal thought usually has the word "I," "me," "my," or "we" in it.

WORKBOOK

Have students answer and correct question #3 on page 6.3.

153

Identifying Negative Personal Thoughts

Group Activity

WORKBOOK   Ask students to look at the Negative Thoughts Baseline on page 5.7.

Which of the negative thoughts you have listed on page 5.7 are *PERSONAL*? Put a checkmark by them.

Leader: Make sure students have put checkmarks next to the statements with "I," "me," "my," or "we" in them.

WORKBOOK   Ask students to turn to page 6.9.

Now list the five or six personal negative thoughts that you feel are the *MOST TROUBLESOME* in the appropriate boxes on page 6.9. Don't list nonpersonal thoughts. We'll work with them later.

Leader: If necessary, students can fill up all of the boxes on page 6.9.

Break (10 min.)

Let's take a *10-minute* break.

IV. CHANGING NEGATIVE THINKING TO POSITIVE THINKING (50 min.)

Objectives
1. To discuss how to use positive thoughts to counter negative thoughts.
2. To provide feedback as students identify irrational beliefs in cartoon sequences and suggest more positive, rational beliefs.
3. To help each student develop positive counterthoughts and beliefs for his or her negative thoughts.

Using Positive Counterthoughts

Negative thoughts can make you feel depressed and unhappy. Positive thoughts make you feel "up" and cheerful. When you think positively about yourself and the world, you feel better. The techniques we're going to learn next have to do with *CHANGING OUR THOUGHTS* in order to control our feelings. The first technique involves the use of *POSITIVE COUNTERTHOUGHTS*.

When you catch yourself thinking negatively, replace the negative thought with a positive "counterthought."

Definition: A *POSITIVE COUNTERTHOUGHT* relates to the *SAME TOPIC* as the negative thought, but it's *MORE REALISTIC* and *MORE POSITIVE*. Negative thoughts and positive counterthoughts have the same sort of relationship between them as "Good News" and "Bad News" stories.

| WORKBOOK | Ask students to read the Herman cartoon on page 6.4. |

1. **What is the "good news" or positive counterthought?**
   (Answer: "He won't be scratching my furniture anymore.")

2. **What do you suppose the "bad news" is?**
   (Answer: "Your pet is dead." This is also the activating event.)

<u>Leader</u>: Ask students to fill in the thought diagram at the bottom of page 6.4. Briefly review the students' answers on the thought diagram.

| WORKBOOK | Ask students to read the Wizard of Id cartoon on page 6.5. |

3. **What is the negative thought in the Wizard of Id cartoon?**
   (Answer: "I have a 105° temperature [I'm sick].")

4. **What is the positive counterthought?**
   (Answer: "The fungus in my cell may dry up.")

5. **Are these two thoughts on the same topic?**
   (Answer: Yes.)

Leader: Ask students to fill in the thought diagram at the bottom of page 6.5.

6. **In these two cartoons (Herman and Wizard of Id), one positive counterthought is more realistic than the other. Which one is it?**
(Answer: "My pet won't be scratching the furniture anymore." Fevers don't really dry up fungi, so this thought is not as realistic.)

7. **What are some positive counterthoughts to the following negative thoughts?**

Negative Thought: "Why do so many bad things happen to me?"
(Possible counterthought: "Last week I saw a man with no legs. I'm relatively lucky.")

Leader: Allow students to come up with some alternative answers.

Negative Thought: "I don't have enough willpower."
(Possible counterthought: "Last week I met my pleasant activities goal.")

Identifying Irrational Thoughts

Many of our negative thoughts are irrational. They are often *OVERREACTIONS* to a situation.

EXAMPLE. **Two different girls, Linda and Julie, both ask their friends to go out on Friday night. Both girls' friends say they can't make it because they have too much work to do.**

Linda feels rejected and thinks, "Because my friend won't go out with me tonight, she doesn't like me, and she will *never* want to go out with me again."

On the other hand, Julie thinks, "Well, my friend is busy tonight, but we can go out some other night. She's still my best friend."

The same situation happened to both girls, but their reactions were very different. It's not *WHAT HAPPENED* but *WHAT THEY TOLD THEMSELVES* about what happened that made the difference in how they felt. One girl's thoughts were irrational, and the other girl's thoughts were more positive and more realistic.

8. **Which girl had the irrational thoughts?**
    (Answer: Linda [the first girl].)

How do you discover irrational thoughts?

The basic approach is to *ARGUE WITH YOUR OWN THOUGHTS*. Instead of blindly accepting that all your thoughts are true, you "argue" or "challenge" just *HOW TRUE* your thoughts really are. If they aren't true, they may be irrational.

Leader: Have students generate challenges to the following examples of irrational thoughts.

EXAMPLE #1
Thought. **"If I don't get a date for Friday night, I'm a total failure *forever*."**
Possible challenge. **"Is this really true? Are you a failure in *everything* if you don't get a date on one particular night? Is it possible that you might get a date sometime in the future?"**

Is this thought irrational?
(Answer: Yes.)

EXAMPLE #2
Thought. **"Either I'm a wonderful person that everyone likes, or I'm a real loser."**
Possible challenge. **"Is this really true? Are there any other possibilities? Could you be somewhere in between? How likely is it that you're neither a loser nor everybody's best friend?"**

Is this thought irrational?
(Answer: Yes.)

WORKBOOK	Ask students to turn to page 6.6.

Leader: Have students answer the questions on page 6.6 as a group.

The statements on this page are irrational beliefs. Let's come up with some beliefs that are more realistic to replace them. What are some rational challenges to these statements?

Leader: Solicit ideas for thoughts that are more realistic, and have students write them down in their workbooks.

```
┌─────────────┐
│  WORKBOOK   │      Ask students to turn to page 6.7.
└─────────────┘
```

Let's look at how irrational thinking affects some cartoon characters. These are some examples of irrational beliefs that involve *EXAGGERATIONS*. The cartoon characters notice one wrong thing and then believe that *EVERYTHING* is wrong with themselves or with some other situation. Read the Garfield cartoon at the top of the page.

1. **Do you remember the negative thought for this cartoon?**
   (Answer: "I feel like such an unworthy parent.")

2. **This isn't the *WHOLE* thought. Sometimes there is more to the whole belief that can be discovered just beneath the surface issues. What is the *UNDERLYING* thought that makes this a depressing situation for Garfield's owner?**
   (Answer: "If Garfield has a bad experience just once because I make a mistake, I'm an unworthy parent." Or, "I'm TOTALLY RESPONSIBLE for what happens to my cat. Even if he's the one who chooses to watch TV, I'm responsible for the consequences. I must always do everything for my cat.")

Leader: Ask students to fill in the Activating Event and Belief boxes on page 6.7.

3. **How can we argue with this belief?**
   (Answer: Accept the ideas offered by students for arguing with this belief.)

4. **What is a more positive counterthought that would be more rational?**
   (Possible answer: "This was a bad experience for Garfield. I'll have to remember to send him to bed and make sure the TV is turned off next time.")

Leader: Ask students to fill in the box for Positive Counterthoughts on page 6.7.

Another category of irrational beliefs is having *UNREASONABLE EXPECTATIONS* of someone else. An example of this type of belief is "I'm embarrassed that my parents don't drive a Mercedes."

Small Group Activity

Leader: Do this activity *only if there is sufficient time.*

WORKBOOK	Ask students to turn to page 6.8.

Have students divide into small groups, and ask them to work together to fill in the thought diagrams for the Cathy cartoon on page 6.8. If the task is too difficult for the students to do in small groups, have everyone work together as a whole group. Help the students arrive at something similar to the following conclusions.

Irrational Belief (Unreasonable Expectation)
"If my boyfriend doesn't think the way I expect him to, his brain is warped, he's bizarre, not normal, etc."

Positive Counterthought
"My boyfriend and I don't agree on this. Each person is entitled to his or her own opinion."

Changing Your Negative Thoughts

WORKBOOK	Ask students to turn to page 6.9.

Look at your list of negative personal thoughts, and write a positive counterthought for as many of them as you can.

Leader: Encourage students to help each other think of positive things about each other. Have them share some negative thoughts and positive counterthoughts to make sure they can apply the skill. Time limit: *5 minutes.*

WORKBOOK	Ask students to turn to the Session Goal Record on page 1.2.

Your goal for this session is to catch yourself thinking negatively at least once every day, then try to change that thought to a positive one. Write this as your goal for Session 6.

V. CONTRACT (5 min.)

Objective

1. To help each student write a contract and select a reward for meeting his or her negative thinking goal.

WORKBOOK	Ask students to turn to page 6.10.

At the bottom of page 6.10 there's a tracking form to help you record negative thoughts and whether you were able to replace them with positive counterthoughts. You will need to fill out this tracking form every day.

At the top of the page, there's a contract similar to the one we used for pleasant activities. I want you to take a minute to fill in the blanks on the contract. Remember, *WHEN YOU CHOOSE A REWARD IT SHOULD BE SOMETHING YOU ENJOY, UNDER YOUR CONTROL, POWERFUL, AND IMMEDIATELY AVAILABLE.*

VI. HOMEWORK ASSIGNMENT (5 min.)

WORKBOOK	Ask students to turn to the homework assignment on page 6.11.

1. Try to meet your main goal for this session, which is to catch yourself thinking negatively at least once each day and then change that thought to a positive one. Use the tracking form at the bottom of page 6.10 to record negative thoughts and positive counterthoughts. Give yourself the reward described in your contract when you are successful in changing a negative thought to a positive one.

2. You also need to keep filling out the Negative Thoughts Baseline on page 5.7.

3. Continue to fill out your Mood Diary on page 1.1.

4. Work on meeting your goal for pleasant activities (page 4.6). You don't have to record the activities, but try to keep doing them.

5. Remember to practice the Jacobsen Relaxation Technique.

Are there any questions?

Success Activity

Let's do our homework for today.

1. If you have already changed a negative thought to a positive counterthought today, check the appropriate boxes on the tracking form on page 6.10.

2. Write down on page 5.7 the worst negative thought you have had today, and record the activating event for that thought.

3. Fill out your Mood Diary for today.

Preview the Next Session

Next session, we'll learn more about getting rid of our irrational thinking.

VII.   QUIZ (5 min.)

| WORKBOOK | Ask students to take the quiz on the power of positive thinking on page 6.12. |

<u>Leader</u>: After everyone has finished, read the answers out loud and have each student correct his or her own quiz.

SESSION 6 QUIZ
The Power of Positive Thinking

1. Which of the following are personal thoughts?

    _____ "I don't have any money."

    _____ "George is a freak."

    _____ "Mary is fantastic."

    ✓ "I'm not too bad myself."

    ✓ "We need to talk."

1 pt. each

2. Write a positive counterthought for each of the following thoughts:

    "I can't run as fast as the other teenagers."

1 pt.   e.g., " But there are other things I can do just as well, or better."

    "My clothes aren't as nice as everyone else's."

1 pt.   e.g., " But my friends like me anyway."

3. Which of the following beliefs are irrational?

    ✓ "All of my problems are someone else's fault."

    _____ "Sometimes I make mistakes, other times I do things right."

    _____ "There are some things I'm pretty good at, other things I don't do so well."

    ✓ "If I don't dress like everyone else in school, no one will like me."

1 pt. each

4. Positive counterthoughts make you feel _____ than the original negative thoughts.

    a. worse
    (b.) better
    c. just the same

1 pt.

162

SESSION 7
Disputing Irrational Thinking

Materials needed for this session:
1. Extra workbooks.
2. Extra pens and pencils.
3. Refreshments for the break.

BLACKBOARD

AGENDA

I. HOMEWORK REVIEW (15 min.)

II. DISCOVERING IRRATIONAL BELIEFS (20 min.)

III. CONVERTING NONPERSONAL THINKING TO PERSONAL THINKING (10 min.)

Break (10 min.)

IV. THE C-A-B METHOD (40 min.)

V. OTHER WAYS TO DEAL WITH ACTIVATING EVENTS (15 min.)

VI. HOMEWORK ASSIGNMENT (5 min.)

VII. QUIZ (5 min.)

RULE: Your beliefs can change how you feel.

I.   HOMEWORK REVIEW (15 min.)

Before I present any new material, let's quickly review some of the ideas that have been presented in previous sessions. I'm going to ask some questions—please raise your hand if you think you know the answer.

Oral Review/Quiz

1.   **What are two characteristics of a positive counterthought?**
     (Answer: It relates to the same topic as the negative thought, but it's more realistic.)

2.   **How does a negative thought make you feel?**
     (Answer: Depressed, nervous, scared.)

3.   **How does a positive thought make you feel?**
     (Answer: Happy and more self-confident.)

4.   **What is the first thing we should always look for when we analyze our thinking?**
     (Answer: The Activating Event.)

5.   **Can we control our thinking?**
     (Answer: Yes.)

Review Student Progress/Record Forms

<u>Leader</u>: Keep the review moving along. The time limit for each question is *1 to 2 minutes*.

A.   **Session Goal (page 1.2)**

  1.   **Did you catch yourself thinking negative thoughts? Did you write them down on page 5.7 and record them on page 6.10?**
  2.   **Were you able to change the negative thoughts to positive counterthoughts? Would anyone care to offer some examples?**

3.   Were you able to do this at least once every day? Did you reward yourself when you were successful?

B.   **Mood Monitoring (page 1.1)**

1.   Did you remember to fill out your Mood Diary every day?
2.   Have you noticed any improvement in your mood?

C.   **Pleasant Activities** (optional)

1.   Did you try to maintain your level of pleasant activities?
2.   Do you need to continue monitoring yourself to keep your pleasant activities level at or above your goal (page 4.6)?

D.   **Social Skills** (optional)

1.   Have you had opportunities to practice your social skills? Did you go to any parties? Did you meet any new people?
2.   Are you enjoying social activities more?

E.   **Relaxation** (optional)

1.   Have you practiced the Jacobsen Relaxation Technique lately?

Group Activity

<u>Leader</u>: Guide students through a brief, *5-minute* relaxation exercise using the guidelines in Session 3.

II.   DISCOVERING IRRATIONAL BELIEFS (20 min.)

Objective
1.   To identify the irrational beliefs in cartoon sequences and replace them with positive counterthoughts.

Irrational Beliefs and Positive Counterthoughts

Last session, we identified some irrational thoughts in cartoon sequences. These irrational thoughts had to do with exaggerations and expectations of others. Let's practice that again.

It's often easier to recognize irrational thinking when we can identify the whole thought. *THE WHOLE THOUGHT IS CALLED THE BELIEF*. The rule for this session is that your beliefs can change how you feel.

WORKBOOK   Ask students to look at the Cathy cartoon on page 7.1.

Leader: Have students identify the activating event and irrational belief in the Cathy cartoon. Then ask them to replace the irrational belief with a positive counterthought. Have students write their answers in the appropriate boxes at the bottom of the page.

Correct and compare answers. The boxes should be filled in approximately as follows:

Answers

Cathy (page 7.1)

> *ACTIVATING EVENT:* Irving is spending money on some faddish things.
> *IRRATIONAL BELIEF:* "If Irving really loved me, he would spend his money on me, his girlfriend, instead of on faddish stuff for himself."
> *POSITIVE COUNTERTHOUGHT:* "Irving has the right to spend his money on whatever he wants; it doesn't mean he loves me any less."

Another common type of irrational belief is jumping to conclusions. An example of this type of irrational belief is "If I look and act like everyone else my age I'll be popular, and being popular will make me happy."

WORKBOOK   Ask students to look at the Garfield and Spiderman cartoons on pages 7.2 and 7.3, and ask them to complete the worksheets.

Leader: Page 7.3 is optional, depending on how much time you have and how well the group seems to be understanding the concepts.

Correct and compare answers after the students complete the worksheets on both pages. The answers should be approximately as follows:

Answers

Garfield (page 7.2)

ACTIVATING EVENT: Garfield has to go somewhere with his "parent."

IRRATIONAL BELIEF: "I'm ashamed to be seen doing anything with my parents because everyone thinks it's dumb to do things with their parents, and I can never do anything that everybody thinks is dumb."

POSITIVE COUNTERTHOUGHT: "It doesn't matter what I do, as long as it doesn't hurt anybody, including myself."

Spiderman (page 7.3)

ACTIVATING EVENT: Spiderman told MJ his secret.

IRRATIONAL BELIEF: "MJ should fall into my arms, hopelessly in love, when she finds out my true identity."

POSITIVE COUNTERTHOUGHT: "I don't know how MJ will react. She may be shocked or need some time to adjust to my true identity."

III. CONVERTING NONPERSONAL THINKING TO PERSONAL THINKING (10 min.)

Objective

1. To help each student convert nonpersonal thinking to personal thinking by identifying the activating event and describing his or her personal reaction to it.

Finding the Personal Belief "Behind" Nonpersonal Negative Thoughts

Sometimes when we react to a particular activating event, we have a negative thought that involves someone or something else, but not ourselves. Here's an example.

BLACKBOARD

> **Activating Event**
>   Getting poor grades at school.
>
> **Nonpersonal Belief**
>   "School sucks! I have bad
>   teachers!"
>
> **Consequences**
>   Getting mad, angry, upset, or
>   maybe depressed.

If nonpersonal thoughts make us feel down, they may be *PERSONAL THOUGHTS IN DISGUISE*. Last session, we looked at our personal negative thoughts. Now we're going to look at nonpersonal negative thoughts to see why they make us feel negative or down. We're going to remove the disguise from these thoughts to see what personal thoughts are behind them.

We can use the A-B-C method with our thought diagrams to do this. These are the three steps.

BLACKBOARD

> 1. Identify the <u>A</u>ctivating event.
> 2. Define the <u>B</u>elief.
> 3. Notice the <u>C</u>onsequences; that is, how the event makes you feel.

WORKBOOK   Ask the students to look at the Calvin & Hobbes cartoon sequence on page 7.4.

Let's work on the Calvin & Hobbes cartoon together. I want you to fill out the thought diagram as we discuss the cartoon.

1. **What is the nonpersonal negative thought?**
    (Answer: "You never let me do anything.")

2. **Identify the activating event.**
    (Answer: Calvin's mom won't let him drive the car.)

3. **What is the disguised personal belief?**
    (Answer: "Just because I'm young, you think that I'm not skilled or responsible enough to drive the car.")

4. **What would be a more rational way to think (positive counterthought)?**
    (Answer: "It's illegal for me to drive the car right now, but mom will let me drive when I'm old enough.")

Look at Your Own Nonpersonal Negative Thinking

You might have nonpersonal negative thoughts such as "Fred is a jerk" or "Sally is rude" or "School sucks." These thoughts are the result of some activating event or events. If you can identify the event that caused this thinking, you can uncover the hidden personal thought.

For example, Fred might have failed to do something you expected him to do in a certain situation. The next step is for you to consider whether your expectation was irrational.

WORKBOOK   Ask students to look at the thought diagrams on pages 7.5 and 7.6.

Choose two of the nonpersonal thoughts that you listed on page 5.7 (Negative Thoughts Baseline). Write one of them at the top of page 7.5, and write the other one at the top of page 7.6. Then fill in the thought diagram on both pages.

Session 7

Leader: Have students work on page 7.6 later if there isn't enough time to do it now.

Break (10 min.)

Let's take a *10-minute* break.

IV. USING THE C-A-B METHOD (40 min.)

Objective

1.   To demonstrate how to analyze negative feelings using the C-A-B approach.

When we're depressed, we often aren't aware of what is making us feel that way. In this situation, the C-A-B method is a useful technique for analyzing our feelings.

The C-A-B method is similar to what we have been doing. The difference is that we start by discovering our depressed feeling (the *C*onsequence), and work from there. Here's a diagram that will help you understand the C-A-B method.

BLACKBOARD

2	3	1
A (*A*ctivating Event)	**B (*B*elief)**	**C (*C*onsequence)**

The Three Steps

1.   **The first step is to notice the *C*onsequence.**

The *CONSEQUENCE* is what prompts us to take action. We notice that we're upset or depressed, and we want to change the situation. The consequence is the emotional *RESULT* of some event or thought.

2.   **The second step is to identify the *A*ctivating Event.**

Then we look at what has happened to find out what's affecting us. This can be difficult. *THE ACTIVATING EVENT* is the situation that "triggers" the depression.

EXAMPLE. Bill and Steve live across the street from each other. Bill feels depressed, while Steve feels happy. What are the emotional consequences for Bill and Steve?

Leader: Write the answers offered by students on the blackboard.

BLACKBOARD

A	B	C
		Depression (Bill)
		Happiness (Steve)

Bill and Steve both look out the window. It's October, and it's raining again. They both notice that the rain affects their feelings.

What is the *Activating Event* for Bill and Steve?

Leader: Write the answers offered by students on the blackboard.

BLACKBOARD

A	B	C
October rain		Depression (Bill)
October rain		Happiness (Steve)

Notice that the same activating event resulted in different consequences for Bill and Steve.

3. The third step is to determine the *B*eliefs that led from the activating event to the consequences.

This is often the most difficult step. To find the beliefs, you must ask yourself, "What was going on in my head when I was feeling depressed?"

[*Note:* The following example was adapted from Kranzler, Gerald. *You can change how you feel.* Eugene, OR: RETC Press, 1974.]

EXAMPLE. It's October and it's raining again. Bill looks out the window and thinks to himself, "This is awful! Summer is over and now it's going to rain nonstop for six months! I can't stand the clouds and the cold! This is horrible! I'll *never* have any fun now!"

Across the street, Steve is looking out his window. He is thinking to himself, "This is great! When it's raining here, that means it's snowing in the mountains. I'll be skiing again soon! I can't wait!"

What are Steve's and Bill's beliefs?

<u>Leader</u>: Write their beliefs on the blackboard.

BLACKBOARD

A	B	C
October rain	"The rain means I can't have any fun for six months."	Depression (Bill)
October rain	"The rain means I'll be skiing soon."	Happiness (Steve)

What actually caused the different consequences for Steve and Bill?
(Answer: Their different beliefs.)

<u>Leader</u>: If students suggest that Steve can ski and Bill can't, indicate that for this example they both know how to ski; the only difference is how they interpret the rain.

Let's review the three steps in the C-A-B Method.

1. **What is the first step?**
   (Answer: Notice the feeling or Consequence—depression, anger, guilt, happiness, etc.)

2. **What do we do next?**
   (Answer: Identify the Activating Event.)

3. **What do we do last?**
   (Answer: Determine the Belief that led to the Consequence.)

The next step is to *ARGUE WITH YOURSELF* to decide whether the belief is irrational. We have already practiced this. Ask yourself, "Are there other ways to look at the situation? What are some other possibilities?"

4. **How can you recognize irrational beliefs?**
   (Answer: They are often EXAGGERATIONS, UNREALISTIC EXPECTATIONS of yourself or someone else, or they involve JUMPING TO CONCLUSIONS.)

<u>Leader</u>: Students should focus on the difference between rational and irrational beliefs. Avoid giving a detailed explanation of the differences between exaggerations, unrealistic expectations, and jumping to conclusions.

5. **Look at Bill's beliefs. What is irrational about them? Why?**
   (Answer: Bill is EXAGGERATING how bad it will be: "This is horrible!" He is also OVERGENERALIZING: "I'll never have any fun now!")

Now we can replace the irrational beliefs with a positive counterthought that's more realistic.

6. **What are some positive counterthoughts that would help Bill look forward to winter even if he can't ski?**
   (Possible answers: He could focus on the fact that hunting season is coming up, basketball season is starting, etc.)

| WORKBOOK | Ask students to look at the Spiderman cartoon on page 7.7. |

Let's read the Spiderman cartoon together. Then we'll analyze it using the C-A-B method.

Leader: After reading the cartoon, ask students to identify the consequence, the activating event, and the irrational belief. Then have them suggest some positive counterthoughts that could replace the irrational belief.

Answers

Spiderman (page 7.7)

CONSEQUENCE: Spiderman feels lonely, guilty, and overly responsible.
ACTIVATING EVENT: Keeping his identity a secret.
IRRATIONAL BELIEF: "Because my aunt worries about my sleeping, eating, and keeping warm, she could never cope with knowing who I am, so I can never tell anyone in the world my identity."
POSITIVE COUNTERTHOUGHTS: "I should be honest with people, especially those who love me. My old, frail aunt should be confident that I am big and strong and I can take care of myself."

V. OTHER WAYS TO DEAL WITH ACTIVATING EVENTS (15 min.)

Objectives
1. To present five ways to deal with activating events.
2. To have students determine the best way to handle activating events in cartoons and other examples.

There are five ways we can deal with activating events.

BLACKBOARD

> 1. Don't respond to them.
> 2. Change the way we respond to them.
> 3. Avoid them.
> 4. Change them.
> 5. Cope with them.

In Session 9, we'll learn some thought interruption techniques that will help us *NOT RESPOND* to activating events.

We have already learned how to *CHANGE* the way we respond to activating events by using the A-B-C and C-A-B methods.

We can also simply *AVOID* activating events. How can we do this?
(Answer: Schedule time to avoid problem situations, make clear decisions in advance about the people you want to spend time with, and study or make other necessary preparations in order to avoid stressful or negative situations such as failing tests, etc.)

<u>Leader</u>: Ask students to offer some specific examples.

In later sessions, we'll be learning new skills to help us *CHANGE* activating events, and we'll discuss some methods for *COPING* with them. These include improving our communication skills and using problem-solving techniques. The Jacobsen Relaxation Technique that we have been practicing can be used to cope with unavoidable activating events and reduce the impact they have on our mood.

WORKBOOK

Ask students to look at the examples on page 7.8.

On page 7.8, there are examples of some problems you might encounter when you use the C-A-B method to change your thinking. Decide which of the five ways to deal with activating events would be best to use in each of these examples.

<u>Leader</u>: Time limit: *2 or 3 minutes.*

WORKBOOK

Ask students to look at the Peanuts cartoon on page 7.9.

Read the Peanuts cartoon on page 7.9, then fill in the thought diagram for Peppermint Pattie.

<u>Leader</u>: When 80% of the students have finished, compare and correct answers.

Answers

Peanuts (page 7.9)

   CONSEQUENCE: **Peppermint Pattie feels incompetent, frustrated, and angry with herself.**
   ACTIVATING EVENT: **Receiving a D-minus.**
   BELIEF (WHOLE THOUGHT): **"A D-minus is a terrible grade. This means I'm a total failure, and I'll never be able to get good grades like everyone else."**
   POSITIVE COUNTERTHOUGHT: **"The D-minus I got on this test (or assignment) is only a small part of what determines the final grade I'll receive in this class. I'll do better next time. And even if I don't do very well in this class, there are other things that I'm good at, so I'm not a total failure."**

WORKBOOK	If there is enough time, have students fill in the thought diagram for the dark-haired girl on page 7.10.

Answers

Peanuts (page 7.10)

   CONSEQUENCE: **The dark-haired girl feels incompetent, frustrated, and angry with herself.**
   ACTIVATING EVENT: **Receiving a B-plus.**
   BELIEF (WHOLE BELIEF): **"A B-plus is a terrible grade. This means I didn't live up to my usual standards, and I'm a total failure. I'll never be able to get good grades again."**
   POSITIVE COUNTERTHOUGHT: **"Most people would consider a B-plus to be a good grade. It means I did better on the test (or assignment) than almost everyone else. I know I can do better next time, and I can still get an A in the class."**

WORKBOOK	If there is enough time, have students turn to page 7.11.

Answer question #1 at the top of the page, then read the Shoe cartoon. Think about the way that the cartoon characters deal with the activating events.

Leader: Discuss some ways to deal with the activating event in the cartoon, and try to come to a consensus regarding which approach would be best. A combination of choices is also a possibility. Time limit: *5 minutes.*

WORKBOOK	Ask students to turn to page 7.12.

Now I want you to analyze one of your own situations. Think of a time this week when you were feeling down. Use the C-A-B method to diagram the situation. Replace your irrational beliefs with positive counterthoughts that are more realistic.

If you decide that your beliefs aren't irrational, then determine which course of action would be best for you. We'll learn how to cope with events and possibly change them in later sessions.

VI. HOMEWORK ASSIGNMENT (5 min.)

WORKBOOK   Ask students to turn to the homework assignment on page 7.13.

1. Try to meet your session goal, which is to analyze a personal situation by using the C-A-B method and filling out a thought diagram once each day (there are four copies of the thought diagram in your workbook on pages 7.15 through 7.18). Write this on your Session Goal Record (page 1.2).

2. Keep recording negative thoughts and positive counterthoughts on page 6.10. Remember to give yourself the larger reward specified in your contract if you achieve your goal five days out of seven.

3. Continue to fill out your Mood Diary (page 1.1).

4. Work on meeting your goal for maintaining a satisfactory level of pleasant activities.

5. Remember to keep using the Jacobsen Relaxation Technique.

Are there any questions?

Success Activity

Fill out your Mood Diary for today.

Preview the Next Session

Next session, we'll learn another relaxation technique.

VII.   QUIZ (5 min.)

| WORKBOOK | Have students take the quiz on disputing irrational thinking on page 7.14. |

<u>Leader</u>: After everyone has finished, read the answers out loud and have each student correct his or her own quiz.

SESSION 7 QUIZ
Disputing Irrational Thinking

1. Think of a personal thought that could be behind the nonpersonal thought below.

   Nonpersonal thought: "You're a jerk."

   Personal thought: <u>e.g., "When I'm around you, and you</u>
   <u>act that way, I feel mad at you."</u>

2. Name three of the five ways to deal with activating events.

   a. <u>(1) Avoid them (2) Don't respond</u> b. <u>(3) Change them</u>

   c. <u>(4) Cope with them (5) Change the way you respond</u>

3. There are two irrational thoughts in the Bloom County cartoon below. Fill in the thought diagram for one of the irrational thoughts.

   BLOOM COUNTY   **Berke Breathed**

   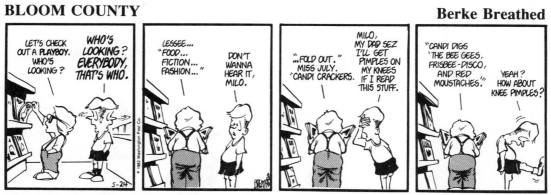

   Bloom County: © 1982, Washington Post Writers Group. All rights reserved. Reprinted by permission.

   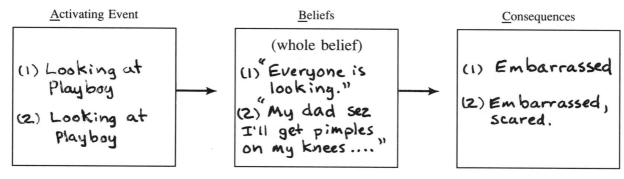

<u>A</u>ctivating Event	<u>B</u>eliefs	<u>C</u>onsequences
(1) Looking at Playboy (2) Looking at Playboy	(whole belief) (1) "Everyone is looking." (2) "My dad sez I'll get pimples on my knees...."	(1) Embarrassed (2) Embarrassed, scared.

179

SESSION 8
Relaxation

Materials needed for this session:
1. Extra workbooks.
2. Extra pens and pencils.
3. Refreshments for the break.
4. Finger thermometers and masking tape.

BLACKBOARD

AGENDA
- I. HOMEWORK REVIEW (10 min.)
- II. C-A-B PRACTICE (10 min.)
- III. IMPROVING FRIENDLY SKILLS (20 min.)
- IV. USING RELAXATION TECHNIQUES EFFECTIVELY (10 min.)
  Break (10 min.)
- V. THE BENSON RELAXATION TECHNIQUE (35 min.)
- VI. THE QUICK BENSON (10 min.)
- VII. HOMEWORK ASSIGNMENT (10 min.)
- VIII. QUIZ (5 min.)

RULE: A relaxed person is a happy person.

I.   HOMEWORK REVIEW (10 min.)

Let's begin by reviewing some of the ideas we have covered in previous sessions. I'm going to ask some questions—please raise your hand if you think you know the answer.

Oral Review/Quiz

1. **What is the A-B-C method for diagraming your thoughts?**
    (Answer: Identify the Activating event, the Belief [whole thought], and the the Consequence [emotional reaction].)

2. **What is the C-A-B method?**
    (Answer: Notice the feeling FIRST, then identify the activating event, and determine the thought that led to the feeling.)

3. **Which method is best when you know you're depressed, but you don't know why?**
    (Answer: The C-A-B method, because you start with how you feel.)

4. **What does the "A" stand for?**
    (Answer: The Activating event, which is the specific situation or event that triggered the feeling or reaction.)

5. **What does the "B" stand for?**
    (Answer: The Belief, which is the whole thought.)

6. **What does the "C" stand for?**
    (Answer: The Consequence, which is the feeling caused by the thought.)

Review Student Progress/Record Forms

A. Session Goal (page 1.2)

1. Did you diagram your negative thoughts using the C-A-B forms (pages 7.15 through 7.18)?
2. Were you able to change your thinking about the event fairly consistently?
3. Did you feel differently after substituting a positive counterthought?

Team Activity

Leader: Form teams by grouping students in pairs (or form groups of three if there is an odd number of students). Time limit: *2 minutes* each.

Take turns sharing with your partner one of the thoughts you diagramed this week. Explain the situation and describe how you handled it, before and after diagraming your thought. You may choose a situation you found difficult to analyze and ask your partner's advice, or you may share a situation you handled successfully. The time limit for each person is *2 minutes*, so you'll need to keep the discussion moving along. I'll give a signal when it's time for the other person's turn. Let's begin now.

Leader: Give a verbal cue at the *2-minute* mark, and reassemble the whole group after *4 minutes*.

B. Negative Thoughts Contract (page 6.10)

1. Did you record negative thoughts and positive counterthoughts?
2. Were you able to meet your goal five days out of seven? If you were successful, did you remember to give yourself the reward specified in the contract?

C. Mood Monitoring (page 1.1)

1. Did you remember to record your mood ratings?
2. Have you noticed any improvement in your mood?

D. Pleasant Activities (optional)

1. Were you able to meet your goal for pleasant activities (page 4.6)?

E. Relaxation (optional)

1. **Have you used the Jacobsen Relaxation Technique lately? Did it seem to work?**

F. Social Skills (optional)

1. **Did you have any opportunities to practice social skills?**
2. **Did you go to any parties?**
3. **Did you meet any new people?**

II. C-A-B PRACTICE (10 min.)

Objective

1. To practice using the C-A-B method by analyzing a cartoon sequence.

WORKBOOK	Ask students to turn to pages 8.1 and 8.2.

Look at the Garfield cartoon on page 8.1. Notice that Garfield has two different feeling reactions in this cartoon.

1. **What are Garfield's two feelings?**
   (Answer: He's happy at first, then embarassed or humiliated.)

2. **Would you use the A-B-C method or the C-A-B method to analyze this situation?**
   (Answer: The C-A-B method would be best, although either method would work.)

Use the C-A-B method to analyze the Garfield cartoon. Since there are two feelings, you will need to use two thought diagrams. Fill in the two empty boxes at the bottom of page 8.1. Then turn to page 8.2 and fill in the two boxes at the bottom of the page.

<u>Leader</u>: When most of the students have finished, briefly discuss the answers.

Answers

Garfield (page 8.1)
CONSEQUENCE: **Happy, "ha ha" feeling.**
ACTIVATING EVENT: **Odie is wearing a dog coat to go on a walk.**
BELIEF: **"Anyone who looks different is funny-looking."**

Answers

Garfield (page 8.2)
CONSEQUENCE: **Feeling humiliated, embarrassed.**
ACTIVATING EVENT: **Garfield is wearing a ridiculous outfit to go on a walk.**
BELIEF: **"Anyone who looks different is funny-looking."**

In this cartoon, two different activating events cause two different feelings as a result of the same underlying belief.

1. **Is the belief irrational?**
    (Answer: Yes.)

2. **What would be a more rational belief?**
    (Possible answer: "Feeling comfortable with the way I look is more important than what other people think.")

III. IMPROVING FRIENDLY SKILLS (20 min.)

Objectives
1. To discuss habits that turn other people off.
2. To have students give and receive feedback on their friendly skills.
3. To help each student identify his or her two most offensive social habits.

Habits that Turn People Off

Answer this question to yourself. Do you generally feel liked by others? If not, it's possible that you do things that "turn people off."

Here is an example of someone who turns people off.

Leader: Use your body to illustrate how Gloria acts as you narrate the example.

Gloria *smiles very little,* and she looks at the floor or at her lap instead of at you. She usually *sits slouched over,* rather than looking interested and alert. She *speaks slowly and softly,* which makes it difficult to listen to her for long. She frequently plays with a paper clip or rubs her hand on her leg while you are talking to her. She often *fails to show interest in people* and gives the impression that she would rather be left alone. All of this makes you feel as if you don't want to be around Gloria. You would rather be with someone who enjoys spending time with you.

WORKBOOK	Ask students to turn to page 8.3.

On page 8.3, there's a list of habits that can be distracting and irritating to other people. Look at this list and think about yourself. Check the habits you think you might have.

Constructive Criticism

It's difficult to look at ourselves and consider how we affect other people. Today we're going to practice giving each other constructive criticism so that we can look at ourselves more objectively.

How do you give someone constructive criticism?
(Answer: First you say something good about the person, then you describe something that could be changed.)

Review Friendly Skills

Remember our four friendly skills? What are they?

<u>Leader</u>: List the friendly skills on the blackboard as students recall them.

BLACKBOARD

> 1. Make eye contact.
> 2. Smile.
> 3. Say positive things.
> 4. Talk about yourself.

Another important rule for conversations is that *EACH PERSON SHOULD SPEND RELATIVELY EQUAL AMOUNTS OF TIME SPEAKING.* Asking questions is a good way to make sure that each person contributes equally to the conversation. Have you ever had a conversation with someone who talked all the time and never let you say anything? How did that feel?

The goal for the first session was to work on a friendly skill. Now we're going to work on friendly skills again.

Friendly Skills Feedback

Team Activity

Pair up with someone you haven't worked with before. Talk to each other about how doing more pleasant activities or analyzing your thinking has or hasn't helped the way you feel. The time limit for your conversation is *3 minutes*. Try to spend equal amounts of time talking, and ask questions to keep the conversation moving. Notice whether the other person's friendly skills have improved. You may want to focus on the skill your partner targeted as a goal for Session 1 (page 1.2), or you may want to look at other friendly skills.

<u>Leader</u>: Give a verbal cue when the *3 minutes* are up.

Now I want you and your partner to give and receive feedback on friendly skills. *FOCUS ON THE SKILLS YOUR PARTNER HAS IMPROVED* since the beginning of the course. We'll do this one at a time. Decide which of you will start, and I'll let you know when it's the other person's turn.

Look at the list of distracting habits on page 8.3. Decide which of these is *THE MOST IMPORTANT HABIT FOR YOUR PARTNER TO CHANGE.* It may be something that's terribly offensive, or something just a little bit bothersome. That doesn't matter, and you're not going to say anything about how offensive it is. You're just going to give each other feedback on *ONE THING* that could be improved.

For example, if your partner doesn't seem to show interest in what you're saying, your comment might be something like "You could show that you are interested in what the other person is saying by smiling and nodding more often." Make sure you express your feedback in a positive way.

> **I'm going to give you a minute or so to give this some thought, and then you and your partner will exchange feedback.**

<u>Leader</u>: Wait about *60 seconds*, then ask if everyone has thought of one thing to say. If so, have them take turns giving feedback.

Allow some time for a brief discussion of how it felt to give and receive constructive criticism. Take steps to soothe any resentment or "bruised egos" resulting from clumsy or insulting feedback.

IV. USING RELAXATION TECHNIQUES EFFECTIVELY (10 min.)

Objective
1. To identify situations in which it is difficult to use the Jacobsen Relaxation Technique immediately before the situation.

Relaxation and Control

> **When we're relaxed, we have more control over ourselves. Having control over ourselves makes us feel happier. The rule for this session is that a relaxed person is a happy person.**

> **We have learned a lot about how to respond in various situations. It's difficult to respond the way we want to when we're nervous or tense, because we tend to get out of control.**

> **Why is it important to be relaxed?**
> *(Answer: So we can be in control of ourselves.)*

Team Activity

<u>Leader</u>: Time limit: *4 minutes.*

> **Pair up again, and identify situations in which you get tense or anxious and have trouble controlling your reactions. Also discuss situations in which it's difficult to use the Jacobsen Relaxation Technique.**

Leader: Ask for some examples of tension-producing situations, and write them on the blackboard. Note that some adolescents may state that they never feel nervous or tense. In these cases, inquire about situations that produce anger, irritability, lack of self-control, and/or sleeplessness. Explain that relaxation techniques can be used to help control these problems as well.

The Jacobsen Relaxation Technique can help us deal with these situations if we do it on a *REGULAR BASIS*. The technique can be particularly helpful if we use it *JUST BEFORE* a tension-producing situation. However, there are times when it isn't possible to go through the relaxation procedure just before a tension-producing situation. After the break, we'll learn a "portable" relaxation technique that can be used in these situations.

When should you use relaxation techniques?
(Answer: On a regular basis, just before tension-producing situations in particular.)

| WORKBOOK | Ask students to answer questions #1 and #2 on page 8.4. |

Break (10 min.)

Let's take a *10-minute* break. Practice your friendly skills during the break, especially the one you need to improve. Keep in mind the feedback you received from your partner.

V.   THE BENSON RELAXATION TECHNIQUE (35 min.)

Objective
1.   To demonstrate how to use the Benson Relaxation Technique.

Leader: Before proceeding, have each student tape a thermometer to the pad of his or her index finger. The bulb of the thermometer should be fastened lightly but securely.

Now we're going to learn a new relaxation procedure called the *BENSON RELAXATION TECHNIQUE*. The Jacobsen technique we learned earlier is for deep relaxation. It also requires a lot of work and concentration. The Benson technique is an easier, *LESS CONSPICUOUS* way to relax.

For this procedure, you need to *CHOOSE A WORD OR PHRASE* to repeat to yourself. This word will help you forget your worries. Some possibilities include the words "one," "relax," "om," etc. Try to choose a word that will make you feel peaceful and relaxed. Which word do you like?

Leader: Ask two or three of the students which word they might use.

Write the word you have chosen as your answer to question #3 on page 8.4.

Now we're going to learn how to do the Benson Relaxation Technique. Here's a list of the *FOUR THINGS YOU NEED TO DO BEFOREHAND*.

BLACKBOARD

> Preliminary Steps
> 1. Find a quiet, restful place.
> 2. Choose a quiet time of day.
> 3. Get into a comfortable position.
> 4. Let go of today's worries.

Let's repeat the preliminary steps out loud.

The procedure for the Benson Relaxation Technique consists of *SIX STEPS*. I want you to answer questions #4 and #5 on page 8.4 while I write these steps on the blackboard.

BLACKBOARD

> 1. Sit quietly.
> 2. Close your eyes.
> 3. Focus on your breathing.
> 4. Say your word as you breathe out.
> 5. Progressively relax your muscles.
> 6. Do this for 10 to 20 minutes, then sit quietly for a few minutes.

In order to use the Benson Relaxation Technique, you'll need to become familiar with the four preliminary steps and the six steps in the procedure itself. These steps will be easier to remember after you have gone through them a couple of times.

```
┌─────────────┐
│  WORKBOOK   │        Ask students to turn to page 8.5.
└─────────────┘
```

We're almost ready to try the technique, but first I want you to record your *"before"* finger temperature and tension level at the top of page 8.5.

Group Activity

<u>Leader</u>: Guide students through the procedure. Model how to breathe out and say the word, then gradually fade to silence. After *10 minutes*, quietly ask them to begin moving their bodies and have them gradually open their eyes. Ask them to record their *"after"* finger temperature and tension level on page 8.5.

Look at your "before" and "after" temperature readings. How did your finger temperature change, and what does it mean? Which technique do you prefer—the Jacobsen or the Benson?

COMMON PROBLEMS

1. *DISTRACTING THOUGHTS.* Simply redirect your attention by focusing on your breathing and repeating your word or phrase.

2. *EXTERNAL DISTRACTIONS.* Try to avoid this problem by finding a quiet place and time.

3. *PHYSICAL REACTIONS AND SENSATIONS.* Small muscle spasms and tingling sensations are normal. These are signs that your body is relaxing. With practice, these reactions will diminish.

It is important to practice consistently. The more you use the procedure, the better it will make you feel. Before we proceed, answer questions #6 and #7 on page 8.5.

VI. THE QUICK BENSON (10 min.)

Objective
1. To help students learn how to use the "quick" Benson Relaxation Technique.

Here's a quick way to do the Benson Relaxation Technique when you're caught off guard by a tension-producing situation.

1. Check the tension level of the muscle group where you tend to hold tension (for example, your neck, back, or chest). Try to relax those muscles.

2. Take a deep breath and exhale slowly while repeating your relaxation word to yourself.

3. Imagine that you're relaxing in your favorite place.

Changing the way you respond in problem situations takes time, patience, and practice. Don't expect the "quick" Benson technique to work perfectly the first time you try it, but you should notice signs that you are gradually making progress.

Question #8 on page 8.5 asks you to describe the quick Benson technique. Please fill this in now.

VII. HOMEWORK ASSIGNMENT (10 min.)

WORKBOOK   Ask students to turn to the homework assignment on page 8.6.

1. Try to meet your goal for this session, which is to practice the Benson Relaxation Technique four times. Write this on your Session Goal Record on page 1.2.

2. **Fill out a C-A-B form when you catch yourself thinking a negative thought or when you start feeling depressed (pages 8.8 through 8.11). Try to do this at least four times.**

3. **Continue to fill out your Mood Diary (page 1.1).**

4. **Work on your goal for maintaining pleasant activities at a satisfactory level (page 4.6).**

Are there any questions?

Success Activity

1. **Fill out your Mood Diary for today.**

2. **If you can remember having a negative thought or feeling depressed earlier today, fill out a C-A-B form.**

Preview the Next Session

Next session, we'll learn more about communication skills. Good communication skills are important for changing situations that can lead to depression. Communication also helps us cope when there is nothing else we can do.

VIII. QUIZ (5 min.)

| WORKBOOK | Ask students to take the quiz on relaxation on page 8.7.

Leader: After everyone has finished, read the answers out loud and have each student correct his or her own quiz.

SESSION 8 QUIZ
Relaxation

1. John asks Kim to go out on a date. She tells him that she can't make it this weekend because she has to go out of town with her parents. John feels embarrassed and depressed. He thinks, "She doesn't like me. I'll never get a girl to go out with me."

   Which of the following are positive counterthoughts to John's negative thought? Write "C" in front of the positive counterthoughts.

   C   a.   I guess she's busy this weekend. I'll try again next week.

   _____   b.   She didn't want to tell me the truth; that was just an excuse.

   C   c.   Well, maybe she doesn't want to go out with me, but there are several other girls who would.

   _____   d.   That was really stupid of me to ask *her* out. She's too good-looking to ever go out with a guy like me.

   C   e.   Well, that seems like a believable reason why she can't go out with me. Maybe I'll try again later.

1 pt. each

2. What is constructive criticism? __First, say something good about the person, then describe something that needs improvement__

2 pts.

3. When are the two best times to use relaxation techniques?

   a.   __On a regular basis__

   b.   __Just before tense situations__

1 pt.
1 pt.

4. When would it be better to use the Benson (portable) relaxation technique, instead of the Jacobson technique (the tense and relax method we learned first)? Write a "B" when the Benson would be best, and a "J" when the Jacobson would be best.

   J   a.   When you want to relax on a regular basis, at home.

   B   b.   Just before you have to make a presentation in front of the class.

   B   c.   When you're getting ready to ask someone to go out on a date.

   J   d.   When you want to relax very deeply and fall asleep.

1 pt. each

194

SESSION 9
Communication, Part 1

Materials needed for this session:
1. Extra workbooks.
2. Extra pens and pencils.
3. Refreshments for the break.

BLACKBOARD

AGENDA
   I.   HOMEWORK REVIEW (15 min.)
   II. TECHNIQUES FOR STOPPING NEGATIVE
        THOUGHTS (20 min.)
   III. COMMUNICATION (10 min.)
   IV. LISTENING, PART 1 (20 min.)
        Break (10 min.)
   V.   LISTENING, PART 2 (20 min.)
   VI. JUDGMENTAL vs. UNDERSTANDING
        RESPONSES (10 min.)
   VII. HOMEWORK ASSIGNMENT (10 min.)
   VIII. QUIZ (5 min.)

RULE: Positive communication builds good
          relationships.

I. HOMEWORK REVIEW (15 min.)

Let's begin by reviewing some of the concepts we have covered in previous sessions. I'm going to ask some questions—please raise your hand if you think you know the answer.

Oral Review/Quiz

1. **What are the four preliminary steps that are required before using the Benson Relaxation Technique?**
   (Answer: Find a quiet, restful place; choose a quiet time; get in a comfortable position; let go of today's worries.)

2. **What are the six steps in the Benson Relaxation Technique?**
   (Answer: Sit quietly; close your eyes; focus on your breathing; say your word as you breathe out; relax your muscles; do this for ten to twenty minutes.)

3. **What are the three steps in the quick Benson technique?**
   (Answer: Try to relax the muscles that are holding the tension; take a deep breath and exhale while repeating your word; imagine that you are relaxing in your favorite place.)

Let's take a minute to do the quick Benson technique right now.

Leader: Offer advice if students seem to need assistance. Time limit: *2 minutes.*

4. **What is the conversation rule about the amount of time each person should talk?**
   (Answer: The time should be shared equally.)

5. **If the other person doesn't say much, how can you get him or her to contribute equally to the conversation?**
   (Answer: Ask questions and look interested.)

6. **What do the letters stand for in the A-B-C method?**
   (Answer: Activating Event, Belief, and Consequences.)

7. **What is a belief?**
   (Answer: The WHOLE thought, the underlying idea.)

8. **What is a consequence?**
   (Answer: A feeling.)

9. **What two ways did we learn to change the consequence (feeling)?**
   (Answer: We can change the belief, and we can change the activating event or how we deal with it.)

10. **What is the relationship between an irrational belief and the positive counterthought?**
    (Answer: They both relate to the same topic, but the positive counterthought is more realistic.)

11. **What kind of thoughts make us feel depressed?**
    (Answer: Negative thoughts.)

12. **What kind of thoughts make us feel happy?**
    (Answer: Positive thoughts.)

Review Student Progress/Record Forms

A. **Session Goal (page 1.2)**

   1. **Did you practice the Benson Relaxation Technique at least four times?**

B. **C-A-B Diagrams (pages 8.8 through 8.11)**

   1. **Did you fill out a C-A-B form when you had a negative thought or felt depressed? How often did you do this? Did it help?**

C. **Mood Monitoring (page 1.1)**

   1. **Did you record your mood ratings?**
   2. **Have you noticed any improvement in your mood?**

D. **Pleasant Activities** (optional)

   1. **Are you meeting your goal for pleasant activities (page 4.6)?**
   2. **Are you enjoying other activities more?**

3. Does life feel as if it's more fun?

II. TECHNIQUES FOR STOPPING NEGATIVE THOUGHTS (20 min.)

Objectives
1. To present three techniques that can be used to stop negative thinking.
2. To help each student select one of these techniques to try out during the coming week.

Thought Interruption Techniques

During the last few sessions, we've been working on ways to counter or argue with negative and irrational thoughts. Here are some additional techniques we can use to interrupt negative thinking.

BLACKBOARD

> 1. Thought stopping.
> 2. The rubber band technique.
> 3. Set aside some "worrying time."

THOUGHT STOPPING. When you're alone and catch yourself thinking negatively, yell "STOP" as loud as you can. Then say, "I'm not going to think about that any more." Gradually change from yelling out loud to thinking "Stop" to yourself. Then you can use the technique in public.

THE RUBBER BAND TECHNIQUE. Wear a rubber band on your wrist and snap it every time you catch yourself thinking negatively. This will help to prevent negative thoughts.

SET ASIDE SOME WORRYING TIME. If you need to think about certain negative things, then schedule a time for it once each week. Make an appointment with yourself for worrying; fifteen minutes should be plenty. Only allow yourself to worry about negative things during that period of time. When you worry, don't do anything else—don't talk, eat, drink, work, or play. Save up your worries during the rest of the week, and only worry about them during this scheduled time.

| WORKBOOK | Ask students to turn to page 9.1. |

At the top of the page, list the three techniques we have just discussed for stopping negative thinking. Then choose the *ONE* you would like to try for the next week. Write this as your answer to question #2. If this technique doesn't seem to work, you'll need to try one of the other techniques on the list. Choose which technique you'll use as a back up, and write it on the second line for question #2.

III. COMMUNICATION (10 min.)

Objectives
1. To discuss the communication process in terms of sending and receiving information.
2. To illustrate nonverbal communication.
3. To introduce the concept of a communication breakdown.

We have discussed how to start a conversation and keep it going by using friendly skills, how to join and leave a conversation with one person or a group of people, how to say positive things to others, and how to provide positive criticism. Now we're going to build on these social skills by looking at how people *COMMUNICATE* with one another. The rule for this session is that positive communication builds good relationships.

1. **Communication involves *SENDING* and *RECEIVING* information. One person talks (the "sender") while the other person listens (the "receiver"). During a conversation, people typically switch back and forth between the roles of sender and receiver as they take turns talking and listening to one another.**

2. **Words are usually part of the communication process, but there are other ways to send information that don't involve words. This is called *NONVERBAL COMMUNICATION*. For example, your tone of voice, facial expressions, gestures, and the way you hold your body all communicate something to the other person.**

Leader: Demonstrate nonverbal communication by acting out some examples (frown while saying "I'm happy" and so on).

3. Sending and receiving information is a delicate process. Sometimes, the person who is listening receives a message that isn't what the speaker meant to communicate. This is what we call a *COMMUNICATION BREAKDOWN*.

WORKBOOK   Ask students to answer questions #1 and #2 on page 9.2.

<u>Leader:</u> *The correct answers to question #1 are **b** and **d**. The correct answer to question #2 is **b**.*

IV. LISTENING, PART 1 (20 min.)

Objective
1. To demonstrate three ways to respond to what someone else is saying: the irrelevant response, partial listening, and active listening.

Three Types of Responses

Now we're going to look at three ways to respond to what someone else is saying. The first one is called the *IRRELEVANT RESPONSE*.

The Irrelevant Response/Team Activity

Get together with one other person to form a discussion team. Then choose a topic and have a conversation about it. You are required to stay on the topic during the discussion, but what you say must be *UNRELATED* to what your partner is talking about. Act as if you didn't hear what your partner has said.

<u>Leader:</u> Model how this is done. Ask a student to make a statement; then comment on the same topic, but make your response totally unrelated to what the student has said. Time limit: *2 minutes*.

1. How did it feel to make a statement and have your partner act as if he or she didn't hear you?
2. How did it feel to ignore the statements made by your partner?

Partial Listening/Team Activity (continued)

Now we're going to demonstrate another type of response called *PARTIAL LISTENING*. Continue your discussion. Listen to what the other person is saying this time, but only for the purpose of changing the topic to something more interesting to you. In other words, you pay *slight attention* to the person who is speaking, then use the information to politely introduce your own ideas into the conversation. You use a *small part* of what the other person is saying, but you take off in a *different direction*.

Leader: Model how this is done. Ask a student to make a statement about him- or herself, and respond with a similar statement about yourself. Time limit: *2 minutes*.

1. How did it feel to have your partner change the subject right after you made a statement?
2. How did it feel to change the subject right after your partner made a statement?

Leader: This might be a comfortable or routine style of responding for some students. Therefore, some students may not see anything wrong with it.

Active Listening

Let's try a third type of response called *ACTIVE LISTENING*. The three rules for active listening are listed at the bottom of page 9.2. I'm going to write the rules on the blackboard.

BLACKBOARD

> Active Listening
> 1. Restate the message.
> 2. Begin with "You feel . . ."
> 3. Don't approve or disapprove.

Leader: Give a more detailed explanation as you write the short version of these rules on the blackboard.

1. Restate the sender's message in your own words.
2. Begin your restatements with phrases like "You feel . . . ," "It sounds as if you think . . . ," or "Let's see if I understand what you're saying . . . ."
3. Don't show approval or disapproval of the sender's message.

Break (10 min.)

Let's take a *10-minute* break.

V.   LISTENING, PART 2 (20 min.)

Objectives
1. To define and practice using active-listening skills.
2. To show students how to use restatements to improve communication. (This is referred to as "paraphrasing" in the literature. Please use the more familiar word "restate" to mean the same thing.)

| WORKBOOK | Ask students to turn to page 9.3. |

Now we're going to practice *ACTIVE LISTENING.* I want you to read the three examples on page 9.3. Each example is a message that has been shared by a different person. There are three responses after each message. Pick the response that's most likely to be used by someone who is following the rules for active listening.

Answers
MESSAGE 1. The correct answer is b. Answers a and c express the listener's views, but they don't restate the sender's message. Answer b begins with "You're bothered . . . ," which describes the sender's feeling.

MESSAGE 2. The correct answer is a. Answer b predicts how the sender will be feeling next week instead of stating how the person feels right now. Answer c is an irrelevant response even though it's about the sender.

MESSAGE 3. The correct answer is c. Answers a and b are replies to the sender's question that change the topic from the sender to the listener. The guidelines for active listening require that you stay focused on the sender's message, as in c.

Team Activity

Form a team again by getting together with another person. This time, one person is going to make three statements while the other person uses active-listening skills to respond. This won't be a discussion like the first two team activities, because active listening means the sender is the only person who introduces any new information. The person who is listening simply focuses on the meaning of the sender's message. Here's how we'll do it.

1. One person makes a *STATEMENT* about him- or herself, about the other person, or about the relationship between the two of you. Try to use a statement that expresses a true feeling, something that has meaning for both of you.

2. The other person actively listens and *RESTATES THE SENDER'S MESSAGE IN HIS OR HER OWN WORDS*. When restating the message, you should begin with "You feel . . ." or "It sounds as if you think . . . ."

Leader: Ask for a volunteer to help role play these two steps. Have the student make a statement, and model how to restate it using active-listening skills.

Decide which of you will go first, and follow these steps for each of the three statements that person makes. Then switch roles, and have the other person make a total of three statements while the first person restates each message. The time limit for this activity is *2 minutes*. Are there any questions? OK, let's get started.

Leader: Reinforce students for their efforts. Don't require expert paraphrasing skills at this point.

1. How did it feel to make a statement and have your teammate restate it?
2. How did it feel to repeat the statement made by your teammate in your own words?
3. When you were the one who was listening, did you find that you had difficulty understanding the message?

4. **When you were the one talking or sending, did you find that the listener didn't receive the message as you intended?**

Leader: Some of the teams will probably encounter communication breakdowns as they go through this activity. Point out that the only reason they were aware of these breakdowns is because the receiver was giving the sender feedback about the meaning of the message. Emphasize that this type of listening gives the sender an opportunity to clarify any misconceptions.

There are many communication breakdowns that go unnoticed in everyday conversations because people generally don't use active-listening skills. Sometimes these *COMMUNICATION BREAKDOWNS LEAD TO CONFLICT*. This is unfortunate because many of these conflicts could be prevented through the use of active-listening skills.

WORKBOOK

Ask students to look at the rule at the top of page 9.4.

Let's read the rule for good listening together. The rule is: "You can speak up for yourself only after you have restated the sender's message to his or her satisfaction." I want you to think about this rule while you answer questions #1 and #2.

*The correct answers for question #1 are **b**, **c**, and **e**. The correct answers for question #2 are **a**, **b**, **c**, and **d**.*

VI. JUDGMENTAL vs. UNDERSTANDING RESPONSES (10 min.)

Objective
1. To explain the difference between judgmental responses and understanding responses.

We have learned that one way to avoid communication failures is for the listener to tell the sender what he or she thinks the message is. This is called an *UNDERSTANDING RESPONSE*. This type of response lets the other person know that you've heard the message, and it encourages him or her to tell more.

Unfortunately, people usually reply to the sender's message with a *JUDGMENTAL RESPONSE* instead. In this case, the receiver tells the sender what he or she thinks of the message by approving or disapproving, agreeing or disagreeing, etc. This type of response tends to make people talk less about how they feel.

| WORKBOOK | Ask students to answer question #3 on page 9.5. |

The answers to part a of question #3 are 1. U, 2. J. The answers to part b are 1. J, 2. U.

An *UNDERSTANDING RESPONSE* lets the sender know that the message has been received accurately and encourages the sender to expand on the message.

A *JUDGMENTAL RESPONSE* tends to make the sender defensive and can lead to arguments.

In the early stages of a relationship, it's important to use a lot of understanding responses. Later in the relationship, judgmental responses are occasionally appropriate.

Leader: Have students answer question #4. *The correct answers are a and b.*

| WORKBOOK | Ask students to answer question #5 on page 9.6. |

The correct answers are c, e, and f.

VII.   HOMEWORK ASSIGNMENT   (10 min.)

| WORKBOOK | Ask students to turn to the homework assignment on page 9.7. |

1.   Your goal for this session is to practice active listening. Write this on your Session Goal Record (page 1.2). Try to restate a sender's message at least once each day. Also take notes on what happened. There is a worksheet for your notes on page 9.9.

2.   **Continue to fill out your Mood Diary (page 1.1).**

3.   **Work on your level of pleasant activities so that it's at or above your goal (page 4.6).**

4.   **Try to practice relaxation using the Benson or Jacobsen techniques.**

Are there any questions?

Success Activity

Fill out your Mood Diary for today (page 1.1).

Preview the Next Session

Next session, we'll learn more about communication. Specifically, we'll learn how to state our negative and positive feelings.

VIII.   QUIZ   (5 min.)

WORKBOOK   Ask students to take the quiz on communication on page 9.8.

Leader: After everyone has finished, read the answers out loud and have each student correct his or her own quiz.

SESSION 9 QUIZ
Communication, Part 1

1. Which of the following describe the "Worry Time" technique for stopping negative thoughts? Check all that apply.

    _____ a. Every time you catch yourself worrying, snap yourself with a rubber band, or pinch yourself.

    ✔ b. Every time you catch yourself worrying, say to yourself, "I don't need to worry about that now, I'll do that during my scheduled Worry Time later this evening."

    _____ c. Every time you catch yourself worrying, shout "Stop!"

    ✔ d. You make an appointment with yourself to worry (for example, from 5 to 6 p.m. every evening), and you worry *only* during that time.

2. You are talking with someone, and you say "I went downtown yesterday, and I saw this great movie where Benji and Godzilla had this huge fight, and they destroyed downtown Tokyo!" Your friend replies with one of the following statements. For each of these statements, indicate whether it is an **IRRELEVANT RESPONSE** (write "**IR**" in the space), **PARTIAL LISTENING** (write "**PL**"), or **ACTIVE LISTENING** (write "**AL**").

    PL a. "Oh yeah? Well, I saw this great TV show, where Spiderman joins forces with Super Chicken, and they open a combination tanning salon and sushi bar, which is just a front for their crime fighting headquarters."

    PL b. "Guess who I saw downtown? Your old friend, Bob! He was asking about you!"

    IR c. "My parents and I got into this argument about whether I could go to the coast this weekend with everybody. What am I going to do if they don't let me go?"

    AL d. "Oh yeah? It sounds like you had a great time at the movies! Tell me about it. Who won the battle—Benji or Godzilla?"

Continued on the next page

207

3. Which of the following are part of active listening? Check all that apply.

1 pt.
each

  ✔   a. Restate the sender's message in your own words.

_____ b. Get up and walk around the room while you talk.

_____ c. Take the lead in picking the conversation topics.

  ✔   d. Begin with remarks such as "It sounds like . . . ."

  ✔   e. Listen to what is being said without indicating that you approve or disapprove of the sender's message.

_____ f. Use lots of hand gestures while you talk.

SESSION 10
Communication, Part 2

Materials needed for this session:
1. Extra workbooks.
2. Extra pens and pencils.
3. Refreshments for the break.

BLACKBOARD

AGENDA
    I.   HOMEWORK REVIEW (15 min.)
    II. STATING YOUR POSITIVE FEELINGS
       (35 min.)
       Break (10 min.)
    III. STATING YOUR NEGATIVE FEELINGS
       (45 min.)
    IV. HOMEWORK ASSIGNMENT (10 min.)
    V. QUIZ (5 min.)

RULE: Self-disclosure helps relationships grow.

I. HOMEWORK REVIEW (15 min.)

Let's quickly review some of the ideas we have discussed in previous sessions. I'm going to ask some questions—raise your hand if you think you know the answer.

Oral Review/Quiz

1. **What is active listening?**
    (Answer: Restating what someone else has said in your own words to make sure you have received the message accurately.)

2. **What are the three rules for active listening?**
    (Answer: Restate the message in your own words; begin with "You feel . . ." or "You think . . ."; don't indicate approval or disapproval.)

3. **Are these responses judgmental or understanding?**

Response	*Answer*
"Oh, come on—you can do it."	*Judgmental*
"You feel tired and want to give up."	*Understanding*

Review Student Progress/Record Forms

A. **Session Goal (page 1.2)**

    1. **Did you practice active listening?**
    2. **Did you practice restating a sender's message at least once every day, and take notes on page 9.9?**
    3. **How did it feel?**

B. Mood Monitoring (page 1.1)

1. Are you recording your daily mood ratings?
2. Have you noticed any improvement in your mood?

C. Pleasant Activities (optional)

1. Are you meeting your goal for pleasant activities (page 4.6)?
2. Are you enjoying other activities more?

II. STATING YOUR POSITIVE FEELINGS (35 min.)

Objectives
1. To discuss how to make helpful personal statements by using the self-disclosure approach.
2. To teach students how to phrase positive feeling statements in the form of an activating event and a personal-feeling reaction (A-C).

Last time, we discussed the idea that communication involves sending and receiving information. We also went through some practice activities to help us develop better listening skills. Today, we're going to work on some skills to help us *TELL ABOUT OURSELVES* and how we feel. These skills are important for several reasons. One reason is that *BY STATING OUR FEELINGS, WE CAN OFTEN CHANGE THE ACTIVATING EVENTS.*

Stating your feelings lets other people know how you have reacted to them so *THEY CAN CHANGE THEIR BEHAVIOR.* This feedback enables others to increase the behaviors that make you feel good and decrease the behaviors that cause you distress. Sharing how you feel is also a good way to *COPE WITH YOUR FEELINGS.*

Self-Disclosure

It's important to use the right approach when you're telling about yourself and the way you feel. Some approaches are more helpful than others. One approach that's particularly useful is called *SELF-DISCLOSURE.* Self-disclosures are *PERSONAL STATEMENTS* that involve telling important things about yourself and/or sharing your feelings with someone else.

1. **What is self-disclosure?**
   (Answer: Sharing your feelings with someone else and/or telling important things about yourself.)

2. **Why is self-disclosure important?**
   (Answer: Because it helps build good relationships with others—it's an important skill for developing close friendships.)

A good self-disclosure statement has two parts. First you describe *HOW YOU REACTED* (your feeling), then you recount *WHAT HAPPENED* (the activating event or reason).

You can use the self-disclosure approach to describe either positive or negative feelings. First we'll focus on expressing positive feelings.

Stating Your Positive Feelings

You can express a positive-feeling statement by saying something like "You make me happy." It's OK to candidly say that to someone, but it's more effective if you use a *PERSONAL STATEMENT* like "*I FEEL* happy when I'm with you."

1. **How could you rephrase "You understand me" as a personal statement?**
   (Possible answer: "I feel understood when I'm with you.")

It can be difficult to describe your feelings. The easiest way to do this is to use "feeling" words like sad, scared, irritated, upset, happy, angry, confused, and pleased.

2. **What are some other words you could use to describe your feelings?**
   (Possible answers: terrified, nervous, quiet, mean, frightened, loving, and depressed.)

Leader: Write the answers offered by students on the blackboard under the heading "Feeling Words." These words will be used later in a practice exercise.

BLACKBOARD

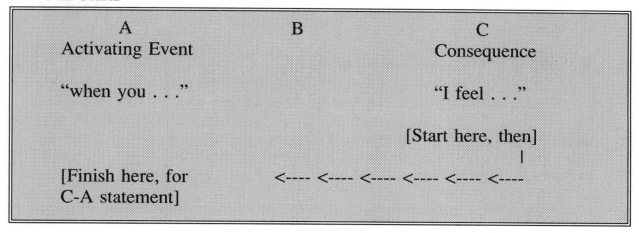

The personal-feeling statement often won't make sense until you describe the reason or activating event. For example, "I'm sad because (situation X) happened." Identifying the activating event also tells the other person why you're feeling that way. This is like our C-A-B method. When we make statements about our feelings, we describe the consequence ("I feel . . ."), and then we identify the activating event ("when you . . .").

Let's illustrate this with an example. It's better to tell someone "I feel warm and happy when you smile" than it is to simply say "You're great" or "You make me feel happy." The first statement is better because it tells the other person how he or she makes you feel *and* it identifies what he or she did to make you feel that way.

| WORKBOOK | Ask students to turn to page 10.1. |

Practice doing this by working on question #1. The question asks you to write some personal-feeling statements you could use instead of simply saying "You make me feel happy." Use the feeling words listed on the blackboard in your statements. Write them in the C-A format that we just discussed—begin with a feeling statement, then identify the activating event.

Now answer question #2 on the same page. I'll give you a minute, then we'll go through the answers together.

a. **"When I'm around you, I feel comfortable and I can be myself."**
(Answer: This is a good personal statement. It's a clear description of how the speaker feels when he or she is with the other person.)

b. **"We all feel that you're really great."**
(Answer: This is not a good personal statement of feelings. The speaker doesn't speak for him- or herself but hides behind the phrase "WE feel." Also, the statement "you're really great" is a value judgment and does not describe a personal feeling.)

c. **"Everyone likes you."**
(Answer: This is not a good personal statement. It does contain the feeling word "likes," but the speaker doesn't state his or her feeling. A personal-feeling statement must include "I," "me," "my," or "mine." Does it seem more caring for a person to say "I like you" or "Everybody likes you"?)

d. **"I feel comfortable in my group."**
(Answer: This personal-feeling statement is a little vague. The speaker begins with the phrase "I feel comfortable," which is the consequence. The activating event is implied, but it's not clearly specified. What does "in my group" really mean? The speaker is implying that there is something about belonging to a group that makes him or her feel comfortable. We can assume that the speaker's positive feeling comes from the acceptance, positive regard, support, and caring that is provided by members of the group.)

e. **"Someone from my group always seems to be near when I want company."**
(Answer: This is not a good personal-feeling statement. The speaker makes a positive statement, but he or she doesn't identify a feeling.)

f. **"I feel everyone cares that I'm a part of this group."**
(Answer: This is not a good personal-feeling statement. In essence, the speaker is saying "I believe" instead of "I feel." The statement describes what the speaker believes other people feel about him or her instead of communicating a personal feeling. The entire statement actually revolves around an activating event, which is being part of a group. The statement could be expanded to make it into a good personal-feeling statement—for example, "I feel accepted and comfortable in my group because everyone seems to care that I'm part of it.")

The rule for this session is that self-disclosure helps relationships grow. This rule emphasizes the importance of self-disclosure, but *WHAT IS THE BEST WAY TO DO IT*? Fortunately, there are some research results that provide answers to this question. We're going to learn how to do self-disclosure the right way.

| WORKBOOK | Ask students to turn to page 10.2. |

Leader: Have students respond as a group to the following statements. Read each statement out loud and ask whether it's true or false. Then give the correct answer and provide an explanation. These are difficult questions and it's easy to answer them incorrectly, so don't let students answer them individually. Encourage some discussion, but limit the time allowed for this. Go through the questions *ONE AT A TIME*, and have students write the correct answers in their workbooks as you proceed.

What Is Helpful Self-Disclosure?

T F **1. Self-disclosure means honestly telling how you feel about what's going on.**
(Answer: This is true. Self-disclosure means sharing with another person how you feel about something the person has done or said about events that have just taken place that you have a common interest in.)

T **F** **2. Self-disclosure means telling *every* intimate detail of your entire life.**
(Answer: This is false. Self-disclosure doesn't necessarily include revealing intimate details about your life. Making highly personal confessions may lead to a temporary feeling of closeness, but a long-term relationship is built by disclosing your reactions to what the other person says and does about events you have both experienced.)

T **F** **3. Hiding your reactions to another person's behavior is a good way to improve your relationship with that person.**
(Answer: This is false. If you hide how you are reacting to the other person, your relationship will not grow or improve. You may be tempted to hide your reactions because you feel ashamed or guilty, or because you want to avoid conflict, or you are afraid of

215

being rejected. But if you cover up your feelings, it can make you seem superficial and insincere, which can lead to social isolation.)

<u>Leader</u>: If students indicate this statement is true, ask them to explain why.

<u>T</u>   F   **4.   Self-disclosure involves risk taking.**
(Answer: This is true. There is a certain amount of risk involved in telling someone how you are reacting to what he or she is doing and saying, but the benefits in terms of building a long-term relationship are well worth it.)

T   <u>F</u>   **5.   When a person's behavior really upsets you, you should reject that person.**
(Answer: This is false. You should describe your reaction to his or her behavior.)

T   <u>F</u>   **6.   Jim meets Mary at a party. Mary immediately begins to tell Jim about her relationship with her father. This is an example of appropriate self-disclosure.**
(Answer: This is false. What Mary is talking about has nothing to do with Jim. See #2 above.)

<u>T</u>   F   **7.   Sandy and Bill are watching a sunset. Bill describes a childhood incident that still affects the way he reacts to sunsets. This is an example of self-disclosure.**
(Answer: This is true. Why? Because Bill's past experience is having an impact on the way he is reacting to something Sandy and Bill are experiencing together.)

T   <u>F</u>   **8.   You should be self-disclosing at all times, in all relationships.**
(Answer: This is false. Your decisions about being self-disclosing should be based on the situation you are in and the nature of your relationship with the other person. A person who discloses too much about him- or herself may scare others away. Being too self-disclosing can create as many problems as disclosing too little. It takes time to build a good relationship, and the level of self-disclosure should be increased gradually as the relationship grows.)

<u>T</u> F   9. **Self-disclosure should be a two-way street—both people in a relationship must participate in the process.**
   (Answer: This is true. One person can take the initiative and encourage the process, but both parties must be self-disclosing for the relationship to grow. The more self-disclosing you are, the more it encourages the other person to be self-disclosing. If you don't respond in a similar way to self-disclosure from another, the other person is likely to stop self-disclosing, and the relationship will stop growing.)

Summary

<u>Leader</u>: Ask students to answer questions #10 and #11 on page 10.2. After everyone has finished, review the answers provided below.

10. **What is self-disclosure?**
    (Answer: Sharing your feelings with someone else and/or telling important things about yourself.)

11. **What is the best way to use self-disclosure statements?**
    (Answer: Make PERSONAL STATEMENTS about your feelings or reactions to the other person's behavior or some shared experience. Both parties should GRADUALLY use them as the relationship grows.)

Break (10 min.)

Let's take a *10-minute* break.

III. STATING NEGATIVE FEELINGS (45 min.)

Objectives
1. To discuss how to express negative feelings by naming the activating event and the feeling reaction.
2. To review the guidelines for making helpful self-disclosure statements about negative feelings.
3. To demonstrate how to use the A-B-C method to sort out problem situations and negative feelings.

Changing Upsetting Activating Events

People often unintentionally do things that upset us. If we tell other people about our negative feelings *IN THE RIGHT WAY*, they are usually willing to try to change the situation. The best way to do this is very similar to the approach we discussed earlier for stating our positive feelings.

We're going to learn how to state our negative feelings to *IMPROVE A SITUATION*. It's helpful to express our negative feelings to the people we care about. If you don't care about the other person, or if you have no desire to improve the relationship, then you should *AVOID THE SITUATION*. The basic rule is "If you don't want to improve a situation, avoid it." Expressing negative feelings in order to make someone feel bad or to get even with him or her is *not* the type of behavior we are practicing here.

We have already learned how to use self-disclosure statements to communicate our positive feelings. Self-disclosure statements can also be used to express our negative feelings and the complaints we have about what other people are doing. It's much harder to state negative feelings, but this is an important skill for building healthy relationships.

WORKBOOK	Ask students to turn to page 10.3.

Leader: Review as a group the pair of negative statements in Part A, and provide a rationale for the correct answer. Then have students answer the five questions in Part B individually. Briefly go over the correct answers when almost everyone has finished.

The second statement in question #5 expresses feelings that probably have been building up for a long time. It's very important to express your feelings as early as you can. A good rule to remember is *"BE HERE NOW!"* If it had been said earlier, the message in question #5 might have been something like "I'm insulted when you tell me I'm too fat in front of other people."

BLACKBOARD

RULE: Be Here Now

It's important to *BE SPECIFIC* when you describe the negative feeling and the other person's behavior that was the activating event or cause. Otherwise, the listener may not understand what he or she has done that upsets you. For example, the statement "I'm mad at you" tells the listener very little about the activating event; it would be much better to say something like "I'm mad because you didn't call me last night as you said you would."

The best approach is to *DESCRIBE WHAT HAPPENED WITHOUT MAKING A JUDGMENT.* If judgments are part of your message, the other person will become defensive and will stop listening carefully to what you are saying. Remember, what you really want is for the other person to hear exactly what you have to say.

GOOD EXAMPLE. "I let you borrow five dollars two weeks ago, and you haven't paid me back yet."

BAD EXAMPLE. "You're a thief and a cheat! You never intended to pay back that five dollars you borrowed!"

If you don't express your negative feelings with words, the message is often communicated nonverbally through body language. It's important to *DESCRIBE NEGATIVE FEELINGS OPENLY WITH WORDS*, especially if you are communicating negative feelings. Body language lets the other person know that you're upset, but it doesn't describe the activating event.

WORKBOOK	Ask students to turn to page 10.4.

Leader: Have students respond to the first item in Part C, then discuss the correct answer and give feedback. Repeat the procedure with each of the remaining items. The following is an outline of the correct answers and points to consider during the discussion.

Write an "F" beside the statements that describe a feeling.

1. ____ a. **"Shut your mouth! Don't say another word."**
   (Answer: Commands like these indicate strong emotion, but they don't describe the feeling prompting them.)
   ____ b. **"What you just said really annoys me."**
   *(Answer: **F**—The speaker states that he or she feels annoyed, and why.)*

219

2. ____ a. **"What's the matter with you? Can't you see I'm trying to work?"**
   (Answer: There are strong feelings behind these questions, but the feelings aren't named.)

   ____ b. **"I really resent your interrupting me so often."**
   (Answer: F—The speaker states that he or she feels resentment, and why.)

   ____ c. **"You don't care about anyone else's feelings. You're completely self-centered."**
   (Answer: This is an accusation that expresses strong negative feelings. Because the feelings aren't named, however, we don't know whether the accusations reflect anger, disappointment, or some other feeling.)

3. ____ a. **"I feel depressed about some things that happened today."**
   (Answer: F—The speaker states that he or she feels depressed, and why; some additional information about what happened to make the speaker feel that way would have been helpful.)

   ____ b. **"What a terrible day!"**
   (Answer: The statement appears to describe what kind of day it has been. In fact, it expresses the speaker's negative feelings without indicating whether he or she feels depressed, annoyed, lonely, humiliated, rejected, etc. Also, the activating event is not specified.)

4. ____ a. **"I'm afraid I'll look dumb if I speak up in the group."**
   (Answer: F—The speaker indirectly states that he or she feels inadequate but fails to name the activating event.)

   ____ b. **"I'll look dumb if I speak up in the group."**
   *(Answer: Be careful! This is very similar to the previous statement. In this statement, however, the speaker indicates that he or she actually **is** inadequate, not that he or she just **feels** that way. This statement reflects a judgment the speaker has made about him- or herself.)*

Making Relationship Statements

When you're having trouble in a friendship, relationship statements can be used to improve the situation. Positive and negative relationship statements help to clarify each person's position and encourage the expression of feelings and ideas that can lead to a deeper, more satisfying friendship.

Relationship statements have an *I* (*ME* or *MY*) and a *YOU* (or *WE*) in them.

Leader: Have students answer questions #5 and #6 in Part D at the bottom of page 10.4. Briefly review the answers, and give feedback when almost everyone has finished. *(The correct responses to question #6 are **a**, **c**, **f**, **h**.)*

Summary

| WORKBOOK | Ask students to turn to page 10.5.
|---|

Read the first statement in Part E. Do you think it's true or false?

Leader: Solicit comments, and give everyone a chance to participate. Then give the correct answer, and provide a rationale. Repeat this process for each of the three statements in Part E. The following is an outline of the correct answers and points to consider during the discussion.

T **F** 1. **The purpose of self-disclosure is to try to make the other person improve his or her behavior.**
(Answer: This is false. Self-disclosure involves giving information about yourself, not giving advice. If you tell someone how you feel, the other person may choose to change his or her behavior, or you may both decide to make some changes in your own behavior.)

T **F** 2. **It's best to wait until several disturbing situations have built up before you discuss them.**
(Answer: This is false. If you let disturbing situations pile up, it becomes increasingly difficult to deal with them. You should express your reaction to something that upsets you as soon as possible so there is no doubt about the activating event and the way it made you feel. For example, the other person would know exactly what you are upset about if you made the following statement, "What you just said is the kind of remark that makes me feel pushed away." If you waited until much later and made the

following statement, the other person would not understand what the activating event was: "You always make me feel pushed away." Remember the rule: BE HERE NOW.)

<u>T</u>   F   **3.   The most helpful way to express your feelings is to describe the other person's behavior that you are responding to and state how you feel.**
(Answer: This is true. The most helpful approach is to describe the activating event, which is the other person's behavior you are responding to, and then state the consequence, which is the way you feel. When you make self-disclosures, it's best to separate the activating event from your reaction. This is the same type of approach we practiced when we used the A-B-C method to examine our thinking. Self-disclosures involving negative statements should relate to ONE specific event. General negative statements about several events are not helpful.)

<u>Leader</u>: Ask students to complete Part F on page 10.5. When almost everyone has finished, go over the answers. *(The correct answers for Part F are as follows: **b**, **h**, and **i** are self-disclosing; **d**, **e**, and **k** are active listening. Note that f is NOT included as an example of self-disclosure because the activating event is not described.)*

WORKBOOK	Ask students to read the Bloom County cartoon on page 10.6.

<u>Leader</u>: Read the following questions and solicit answers from the students.

1.   Who has the negative feeling?
(Answer: Steven.)

2.   Name the negative feeling.
(Answer: He is embarrassed and angry at his mother.)

3.   What is the activating event?
(Answer: Steven's mother walks into the bathroom.)

4.   What is the belief that causes the feeling?
(Answer: "I should have privacy in the bathroom.")

5.   Is the belief irrational?
(Answer: No.)

6. **What are Steven's choices? Which is the best choice?**
   (Answer: Steven should describe the activating event and state how he feels.)

7. **Write on the form what Steven should say.**
   (Answer: "When you come in the bathroom without my permission, I feel that my privacy has been violated." He could also state his belief—that he should have privacy in the bathroom.)

8. **What did Steven do wrong?**
   (Answer: He yelled at his mother. He should have responded in a quiet, serious tone of voice.)

Naming Problem Situations

Now we're going to work on some of our own problems, but we're going to start with the *EASY* ones first; that is, those problems which are recent enough that our negative feelings haven't been building up for very long. Some problems have a long history of deep-seated feelings. Let's save those for the later sessions.

I want you to think of a situation in which it's difficult for you to say how you feel. It could be a problem with any of the following:
1. **Refusing a friend's request.**
2. **Telling a friend about something he or she did that bothered you; for example, not inviting you to a party, lying, or revealing something that was confidential.**
3. **Resisting group pressure; for example, not going to a horror movie you don't want to see, refusing to shoplift, not taking drugs at a party, etc.**

WORKBOOK   Ask students to turn to page 10.7.

At the top of the page, write three or four problem situations that you would like to work on.

Leader: Wait until most of the students have finished writing before proceeding.

1. **Now choose one problem situation from your list. Describe the activating event and your feeling (the consequence).**

2. Next, write down the belief that causes your feeling. Is the belief irrational?

3. What are your choices? Which one will you try?

4. Write your A-C statement.

Team Activity

<u>Leader</u>: Time limit: *2 minutes*.

Pick a partner for this role-playing exercise, preferably someone you haven't worked with very much. Then I want each of you to choose a problem from your list at the top of page 10.7 to role play with your partner. One member of the team will present a problem while his or her partner responds using active-listening skills, and then the other person will take a turn. Here are the rules for each person.

1. The team member who is presenting the problem makes a statement about him- or herself, about another person—a friend, a family member, etc.—or about the relationship between them.

2. The other team member role plays the part of the friend, family member, etc. who is involved in the problem and states in his or her *OWN WORDS* what the presenter has said. This restatement should start out with "You feel . . ." or "You think . . . ."

<u>Leader</u>: Ask the students to offer a statement to use as an example, and model how to respond and role play.

DISCUSSION QUESTIONS

1. How did it feel to make a self-disclosing statement and have your partner restate it?

2. How did it feel to restate the feeling statement made by your partner?

3. When your partner was the presenter, was it difficult to understand his or her message?

4. When you were the presenter, did you find that your partner had trouble receiving your intended message?

IV. HOMEWORK ASSIGNMENT (10 min.)

| WORKBOOK | Ask students to turn to the homework assignment on page 10.8.

1. Your main goal for this session is to practice stating positive feelings using the A-C method. Write on your Session Goal Record (page 1.2), "State a positive feeling each day." Use page 10.10 to record your positive-feeling statements, and try to express the thought to the person involved.

2. Another goal for this session is to use the self-disclosure approach to express at least two negative feelings this week. If possible, try to address the problem situation you selected for the role-playing exercise earlier in the session.

3. Analyze a problem situation or a feeling each day, using the A-B-C forms on pages 10.11 through 10.14. If you find that your belief is irrational, change the belief. If you find that the belief is rational, state your feelings.

4. Continue to fill out your Mood Diary (page 1.1).

5. Practice your active-listening skills.

6. Try to maintain a good level of pleasant activities.

7. If possible, practice the relaxation techniques and use them in tension-producing situations.

Are there any questions?

Success Activity

Let's do some of our homework right now. Fill out your Mood Diary for today.

Preview the Next Session

Next session, we'll learn new skills for negotiation and problem solving.

V.   QUIZ   (5 min.)

WORKBOOK   Ask students to take the quiz on communication on page 10.9.

<u>Leader:</u> After everyone has finished, read the answers out loud and have each student correct his or her own quiz.

SESSION 10 QUIZ
Communication, Part 2

Which of the following are good personal feeling statements (self-disclosures)? Check all that apply.

  ✔   a. "We are all very upset about his behavior in class."

  ✔   b. "I'm excited to see my cousins."

  ____   c. "I feel that everyone should give to charities."

  ____   d. "You make me mad when you forget to pick up after yourself."

  ✔   e. "I was very surprised when you gave me a birthday card."

2. What is an acceptable reason for stating negative feelings about a situation or a person? Pick one answer.

  ____   a. To help someone else realize that they are wrong.

  ✔   b. To improve a situation.

  ____   c. To make someone else feel as bad as you did.

  ____   d. To make sure people realize you're not fooled by their behavior.

3. Bill comes home from school and finds his mother in his room, looking through his dresser drawers. He yells, "You never give me any privacy! Get out of here! I hate you!" Even though Bill states his feelings (and he is obviously quite upset), there might have been a better way for him to tell his mother how he feels about her invading his privacy so that she would be more likely to listen to him. Which of the following statements is the best way for Bill to tell his mother how he feels? Pick one answer.

  ____   a. "You never give me any privacy! Get out of here! I hate you!"

  ✔   b. "Mom, when you look through my dresser, it makes me really angry and upset with you. I feel upset because it seems like you don't trust me!"

  ____   c. "How would you like it if I looked through *your* dresser?"

  ____   d. "It's like you don't trust me! What did you think you were going to find—do you think I'm a drug addict or something? You don't trust me!"

SESSION 11
Negotiation and Problem Solving, Part 1

Materials needed for this session:
1. Extra workbooks.
2. Extra pens and pencils.
3. Refreshments for the break.
4. Some 3" x 5" index cards.

BLACKBOARD

AGENDA
- I. HOMEWORK REVIEW (15 min.)
- II. USING ASSERTIVE IMAGERY (15 min.)
- III. RATIONALE FOR PROBLEM SOLVING AND NEGOTIATION (10 min.)
- IV. BASIC RULES FOR SETTLING DISAGREEMENTS (10 min.)
  Break (10 min.)
- V. DEFINING THE PROBLEM (10 min.)
- VI. PRACTICING PROBLEM SOLVING AND ACTIVE LISTENING (35 min.)
- VII. HOMEWORK ASSIGNMENT (10 min.)
- VIII. QUIZ (5 min.)

RULE: Dealing with minor disagreements prevents major conflicts.

I.   HOMEWORK REVIEW (15 min.)

Let's quickly review some of the important points from last week. I'm going to ask some questions—please raise your hand if you think you know the answer.

Oral Review/Quiz

1.   **What do we call positive- and negative-feeling statements?**
(Answer: Self-disclosures.)

2.   **What are we doing when we use self-disclosure statements?**
(Answer: Sharing feelings, telling something about ourselves.)

3.   **What is a relationship statement?**
(Answer: A statement with an "I" and a "YOU" in it.)

4.   **When are relationship statements helpful?**
(Answer: When we want to improve a relationship.)

5.   **Why do we state our feelings?**
(Answer: It lets other people know how we have reacted to something they have done, it can help to change a bad situation, and it's a good way to cope with our feelings.)

6.   **What is the best way to state our feelings?**
(Answer: By using a C-A statement. Say how you feel [happy, sad, etc.], then describe what the other person did or said that made you feel that way).

7.   **Should we only use C-A statements when we are talking to friends?**
(Answer: No, C-A statements are helpful in many types of relationships.)

8.   **Why is active listening helpful?**
(Answer: It clarifies misunderstandings and makes the sender feel understood.)

230

Review Student Progress/Record Forms

A. **Session Goal** (page 1.2)

    1. Did you write down at least one positive thought each day on page 10.10 using the A-C method?
    2. Did you analyze a problem situation or feeling each day using the A-B-C forms (pages 10.11 through 10.14)? Were you able to change your beliefs and/or feelings?
    3. Did you use self-disclosure statements to express your negative feelings? What were the results? Did the activating event change? Did it become easier to cope with your feelings?

B. **Mood Monitoring** (page 1.1)

    1. Are you filling out your Mood Diary every day?
    2. Have you noticed any improvement in your mood?

C. **Active Listening**

    1. Did you have any opportunities to practice active listening?
    2. Did you make some active-listening responses? How did it work?
    3. Have you tried active listening in situations where someone was expressing a negative feeling to you?

D. **Pleasant Activities** (optional)

    1. Are you meeting your goal for pleasant activities (page 4.6)?

E. **Relaxation** (optional)

    1. Do you use relaxation techniques before stressful situations? Regularly?

F. **Other Skills** (optional)

    1. Have you been participating in more social activities? Are you enjoying social activities more?

Group Activity

Let's practice the Benson Relaxation Technique right now, for *2 minutes*.

Session 11

<u>Leader</u>: Read the steps for the relaxation procedure while the students are relaxing. Use the instructions provided in Session 8.

II. USING ASSERTIVE IMAGERY (15 min.)

Objectives

1. To introduce the concept of assertive-imagery practice, and to help students learn the four steps involved in doing it.
2. To have each student work on a problem situation using assertive-imagery practice.

In the last session, we talked about self-disclosure statements. Even with practice, however, it's difficult to use them in real life situations. It's particularly difficult to make self-disclosure statements at the right time, which is *IMMEDIATELY*. Remember the rule—be here now.

Assertive Imagery

To help us use self-disclosure statements more often, we're going to learn a technique called "*ASSERTIVE IMAGERY*."

It feels risky to disclose to someone else how you are reacting to what he or she has said or done. Often, we're afraid of how the other person will respond. One way to overcome this fear is to do some imagery practice. There are four steps involved in doing the imagery practice.

1. ***MAKE A MENTAL PHOTOGRAPH OF THE SITUATION*** **in which you want to use self-disclosure.**
2. ***CONVERT THE PHOTOGRAPH INTO A MOVIE.***
3. **Include in your movie the moment when you *STATE YOUR FEELINGS*.**
4. ***IMAGINE THE OTHER PERSON'S REACTION*** **to your feeling statement the way you would like it to be. What will the person say and do?**

BLACKBOARD

> 1. Make a photograph of the situation.
> 2. Change it into a movie.
> 3. State your feelings.
> 4. Imagine the other person's reaction.

| WORKBOOK | Ask students to turn to page 11.1. |

Write the four steps for assertive-imagery practice in the spaces provided after question #1 at the top of the page.

Group Activity

Now we're going to practice using assertive imagery. Select one of the problems you listed on page 10.7 during our last session. Think about the self-disclosure statement you need to make to resolve the situation.

<u>Leader</u>: Guide the students verbally through the four steps, then give them *1 minute* to do the assertive-imagery practice.

Why is it important to become good at self-disclosure and active listening?

<u>Leader</u>: Ask students to volunteer answers to this question, and write their responses on the blackboard. Add to their comments until you have listed most of the following points.

BLACKBOARD

> 1. Promotes close, warm relationships.
> 2. Prevents arguments and fights.
> 3. Results in more positive responses from others.
> 4. Allows others to understand you better.
> 5. Helps you overcome shyness.

Review these points, and write the three that are most important for you in the spaces provided after question #2 on page 11.1.

III. RATIONALE FOR PROBLEM SOLVING AND NEGOTIATION (10 min.)

Objective
1. To discuss the importance of problem-solving and negotiation skills.

Interpersonal Conflict

Our next topic is the importance of resolving conflicts and disagreements with friends and family members. We will also learn some essential *PROBLEM-SOLVING* and *NEGOTIATION SKILLS*.

During the last two sessions, we have discussed some guidelines for communication. We have concentrated primarily on how to communicate with friends. This is important because we need to know how to make new friends and how to build healthy relationships.

However, *CONFLICTS OR DISAGREEMENTS ARE BOUND TO COME UP*, even with friends you like a lot. This is normal, so it's important to know how to *SETTLE DISAGREEMENTS* that you have with your friends through the use of problem-solving and negotiation skills. If minor disagreements are not settled, then *MAJOR CONFLICTS* are more likely to occur that are *MUCH MORE DIFFICULT TO RESOLVE*. The rule for this session is that dealing with minor disagreements prevents major conflicts.

Here are some examples of issues that tend to create conflicts between friends:
1. What to do and where to go when going out.
2. Asking for favors, and being asked for favors.
3. Who (or what group of people) to spend time with.
4. Things that are borrowed and not returned; for example, money and music tapes.

Leader: Have students generate a list of other conflicts that come up between friends. Write their suggestions on the blackboard.

THE SITUATION IS USUALLY DIFFERENT AT HOME. You have to be around your parents even when you're not getting along with them, and you depend on them for essential things like food, money, and permission to do things. Because of this, it's particularly important for parents and adolescents to learn how to communicate with one another so they can resolve problems without unnecessary conflict. Many families need to learn new ways to communicate, especially if the old ways aren't working.

Here are some examples of the issues that tend to create conflicts between teenagers and parents:
1. Differences of opinion regarding appropriate behavior, the clothes you are allowed to wear, etc.
2. Where you can go with your friends, and when you have to be home (curfew).
3. The chores you are required to do, such as cleaning up your bedroom.
4. Who your friends are, and how much time you get to spend with them.

Leader: Have students generate a list of other issues that create conflicts between teenagers and parents. Write their suggestions on the blackboard.

IV. BASIC RULES FOR SETTLING DISAGREEMENTS (10 min.)

Objective
1. To discuss the basic rules for successful problem solving.

In all conflicts or disagreements, there is someone who has a *COMPLAINT* about someone else. In your family or group of friends, the person with the complaint may be you, your parents, your friends, or just about anyone.

Leader: Discuss and provide a rationale for each of the following points.

1. *THE PERSON WITH A COMPLAINT HAS THE RIGHT TO BE HEARD AND THE RIGHT TO ASK FOR CHANGE*, regardless of how realistic or unrealistic the request may seem.

2. *LISTENING TO SOMEONE'S COMPLAINT DOES NOT MEAN THAT YOU AGREE OR DISAGREE*, it simply indicates that you're trying to understand what changes the person wants. You can disagree later. *THE FIRST STEP IS TO TRY TO UNDERSTAND THE POINT OR COMPLAINT.*

> | WORKBOOK | Ask students to answer questions #1 and #2 on page 11.2.

What communication skills have you learned so far that would help in negotiation?

Leader: Ask students to volunteer some answers. Give each student a chance to contribute to the discussion. Use subtle prompts to generate the following answers.

1. **Use self-disclosure statements to describe the problem in terms of the activating event and your personal feeling.**
2. **Use relationship statements.**
3. **Use active-listening skills.**

Break (10 min.)

Let's take a *10-minute* break.

V. DEFINING THE PROBLEM (10 min.)

Objective
1. To discuss the rules for defining problems.

Eight Rules for Defining a Problem

The way you define or describe a problem sets the stage for the rest of the discussion. If it's done poorly, it may turn others off or make them angry. A good problem definition states *CLEARLY AND SPECIFICALLY* what the other person is doing or saying that creates a problem for you. The definition should

describe to the other person *WHY* it's a problem. Here are several rules for doing it correctly.

1. *BEGIN WITH SOMETHING POSITIVE.*
2. *BE SPECIFIC.*
3. *DESCRIBE WHAT THE OTHER PERSON IS DOING OR SAYING* that's creating a problem for you (use self-disclosures!).
4. Don't describe the problem in terms of flaws in the other person (for example, "You're lazy!"). In other words, *NO NAME-CALLING.*
5. *EXPRESS YOUR FEELINGS* as a reaction to what the other person is doing or saying.
6. *ADMIT YOUR CONTRIBUTION* to the problem. Accept responsibility for your share even if it's just causing others distress.
7. *DON'T ACCUSE* or blame others.
8. *BE BRIEF.*

<u>Leader</u>: Write the following words on the blackboard as you review the rules for defining problems. Leave this list on the blackboard for discussion during the exercises that follow.

BLACKBOARD

> 1. Begin with something positive.
> 2. Be specific.
> 3. Describe what the other person is doing or saying.
> 4. No name-calling.
> 5. Express your feelings.
> 6. Admit your contribution.
> 7. Don't accuse.
> 8. Be brief.

| WORKBOOK | Ask students to turn to page 11.3. |

<u>Leader</u>: Have the students read the examples on page 11.3, and ask them to write down what's right and wrong with them. Remind them to use the rules on the blackboard. After they have finished, go through the exercise again out loud, asking students to volunteer their answers. Make sure everyone has a chance to respond.

1. **"I know you want me to be safe and that you try to take care of me. My problem is that I want to stay out until midnight on weekends to party with my friends, but my curfew is 11:00 p.m. This bothers me because I have to leave parties early, and I miss out on the fun."**
   (Answer: This is a good definition because it begins with something POSITIVE; it mentions SPECIFICALLY what the other person does that creates the problem; it expresses the presenter's FEELINGS; it's BRIEF; and the presenter takes some RESPONSIBILITY for the problem.)

2. **"My problem is that you are too strict about curfew!"**
   (Answer: This definition is not very good because it ACCUSES the listener of being too strict without explaining what is meant by "strict.")

3. **"My problem is that you are irresponsible about taking care of your room."**
   (Answer: This definition also ACCUSES the listener of being irresponsible without providing an adequate explanation. Ask students to identify other weaknesses.)

4. **"I'm upset about the dust on the floor, the clothes on the bed, and the messy papers on the desk in your room. It embarrasses me when my friends come to visit and they see your room."**
   (Answer: This definition is good because it's very SPECIFIC; it FOCUSES ON BEHAVIOR rather than personality; and it EXPRESSES THE PRESENTER'S FEELINGS. Ask students how the presenter could have handled this better—for example, by beginning with something positive, etc.)

VI. PRACTICING PROBLEM SOLVING AND ACTIVE LISTENING (35 min.)

Objective

1. To involve students in a role-playing exercise in which they practice defining a problem and using active-listening skills.

Now we're going to practice defining a problem and using our active-listening skills. As we discussed earlier, active listening means being nonjudgmental and understanding. In this exercise, we're going to check to see how well one person defines the problem and how well the other person understands what has been said.

Team Activity

<u>Leader</u>: Have students form teams by pairing up. If one of the teams has a third member, have that person give constructive feedback to the other members of the team as they role play (that is, name the rules that are followed).

Here are the instructions for this exercise. I want you to take turns playing the roles of teenagers and parents. Each "teenager" will define a problem, and the "parent" will respond with an active-listening statement. The "teenager" will then tell the "parent" whether the message has been received correctly. If the active-listening statement does not accurately reflect what has been said, the "teenager" will restate the problem and the "parent" will respond again. Continue this process until it's clear that the "parent" understands the problem. Then switch roles with your partner, and repeat the exercise with a new problem definition. This exercise should take about *10 to 15 minutes*.

<u>Leader</u>: After most of the teams have finished, discuss the exercise for *5 to 10 minutes*. Ask students what they experienced, both as the "teenager" and as the "parent." Address any issues you may have noticed as you watched the teams go through the exercise. Remind students to follow the rules on the blackboard.

Now we're going to repeat the exercise, but this time the "parent" will define a problem and the "teenager" will respond using the guidelines for active listening. I want you to form new teams for this exercise by pairing up with different partners. Continue going back and forth until it's clear that the "teenager" understands the problem. Then, switch roles. You have about *10 to 15 minutes* for this exercise.

<u>Leader</u>: After most of the teams have finished, bring the practice session to an end.

As you were participating in these exercises, how many of you looked up at the blackboard to read the eight rules for defining a problem? [Ask for a show of hands.] In the beginning, it's helpful to keep these rules handy so you can quickly review them when they are needed. Over time, you will become so familiar with these rules that you will use them automatically. Until then, however, you will need to write them down and carry them with you.

Session 11

Leader: Pass out 3" x 5" index cards, and ask students to copy the eight rules onto a card. Have them place the finished card in their wallets, purses, notebooks, etc.

VII.   HOMEWORK ASSIGNMENT (10 min.)

WORKBOOK   Ask students to turn to the homework assignment on page 11.4.

1. Your goal for this session is to practice defining problems. Write this on your Session Goal Record (page 1.2). During the coming week, identify several problems that you would like to work on. Then, practice defining them using the rules we have discussed in this session. A worksheet is provided for this on page 11.6. *DON'T TRY TO STATE THE PROBLEM TO OTHER PEOPLE YET!*

2. Continue to fill out your Mood Diary (page 1.1).

3. Practice your active-listening skills.

4. Try to meet your goal for pleasant activities (page 4.6).

5. Practice the relaxation techniques and use them in appropriate situations.

Are there any questions?

Success Activity

Let's do some of our homework right now.

1. Fill out your Mood Diary.

2. If you can think of a problem you would like to work on, write it down on page 11.6. Then define the problem.

Preview the Next Session

Next session, we'll learn how to find good solutions to problems by using a technique called "brainstorming."

AN IMPORTANT REMINDER

<u>Leader</u>: The next three sessions (12, 13, and 14) are intended for groups of adolescents only. The modified versions of these sessions that are used when parents participate in the program are provided in Section III of this manual.

VIII.   QUIZ (5 min.)

| WORKBOOK | Ask students to take the quiz on negotiation and problem solving on page 11.5. |

<u>Leader</u>: After everyone has finished, read the answers out loud and have each student correct his or her own quiz.

SESSION 11 QUIZ
Negotiation and Problem Solving, Part 1

1. There are several steps involved in using assertive imagery. Arrange the items below in the correct order by placing a "1" by the first step, a "2" by the second step, and so on. *Leave out any items that aren't one of the steps for using assertive imagery.*

    2   a. Change the photograph of the scene into a movie.

    _____   b. Dispute your irrational thoughts.

    4   c. Imagine the other person's reaction to your statement of your feelings.

    _____   d. Tense, and then relax your muscles.

    1   e. Make a photograph in your mind of the situation you want to prepare for.

    3   f. State your feelings to the other person in the movie.

1 pt. each

Indicate whether the following statements about defining a problem are true or false.

(T) F   2. In defining a problem, you should start with saying something positive about the other person or the situation.

T (F)   3. In defining the problem, you should describe the other person's role in the problem, but don't talk about your own role in the problem.

T (F)   4. Don't express your feelings during problem definition. It only complicates things.

(T) F   5. Describe what happened that bothered you, and what you think needs to be changed.

T (F)   6. This is a good problem definition: "My problem is that you are too lazy! You make me mad when you don't pick up after yourself."

(T) F   7. Name-calling is not very helpful in defining a problem.

1 pt. each

SESSION 12A
Negotiation and Problem Solving, Part 2

Adolescent Only Version

Materials needed for this session:
1. Extra workbooks.
2. Extra pens and pencils.
3. Refreshments for the break.

BLACKBOARD

AGENDA
- I. HOMEWORK REVIEW (15 min.)
- II. BRAINSTORMING (15 min.)
- III. CHOOSING A SOLUTION (15 min.)
  Break (10 min.)
- IV. IMPLEMENTING AND CONTRACTING (15 min.)
- V. PRACTICING PROBLEM SOLVING AND NEGOTIATION (35 min.)
- VI. HOMEWORK ASSIGNMENT (10 min.)
- VII. QUIZ (5 min.)

RULE: Compromise is the key to reaching mutual agreements.

I. HOMEWORK REVIEW (15 min.)

Let's begin by reviewing some of the concepts that were discussed during the last session. I'm going to ask some questions—please raise your hand if you think you know the answer.

Oral Review/Quiz

1. **What are the four steps for assertive-imagery practice?**
   (*Answer: Make a mental photograph of the situation; convert the photograph into a movie; state your feelings in the movie; imagine the other person's reaction.*)

2. **Why is it important to learn problem-solving and negotiation skills?**
   (*Answer: These are essential skills for resolving complaints and preventing minor conflicts from becoming serious. They help to maintain friendships and harmony.*)

3. **What are the two basic rules for successful problem solving?**
   (*Answer: The person with a complaint has the right to be heard; listening to the complaint doesn't mean that you agree or disagree.*)

4. **What are the rules for defining a problem?**
   (*Answer: Begin with something positive; be specific; describe what the other person is saying or doing; no name-calling; express your feeling; admit your contribution; don't accuse; be brief.*)

Review Student Progress/Record Forms

A. **Session Goal (page 1.2)**

   1. **Did you identify one or more problems that you would like to work on?**
   2. **Did you record the problems on page 11.6, and practice defining them using the eight rules?**

B. **Mood Monitoring (page 1.1)**

  1. Are you remembering to record your mood rating every day?
  2. Have you noticed any improvement in your mood?

C. **Active Listening** (optional)

  1. Did you have any opportunities to practice active listening? How did it work?
  2. Have you tried using active-listening skills in situations where someone was communicating a negative feeling?

D. **Pleasant Activities** (optional)

  1. Did you meet your goal for pleasant activities (page 4.6)?

E. **Relaxation Techniques** (optional)

  1. Did you use the relaxation techniques?

II. BRAINSTORMING (15 min.)

Objectives
1. To discuss the rationale and rules for brainstorming.
2. To practice brainstorming by having students generate solutions to some typical parent-teenager problems.

During the last session, we discussed the importance of problem-solving and negotiation skills. We learned how to *DEFINE PROBLEMS* and how to respond with *ACTIVE LISTENING SKILLS* when someone else states a problem. In this session, we're going to learn *NEGOTIATION SKILLS* that will help us resolve issues by working with the other person to reach a mutual agreement.

After the problem has been *DEFINED* so that everyone understands what it is, the next step is to come up with a variety of *DIFFERENT SOLUTIONS* to the problem. At this stage, it's important to be creative and nonjudgmental. Don't be too hasty. Remember, none of the solutions to these problems has worked so far. The more ideas that everyone generates, the better. We call this approach *BRAINSTORMING*.

While there are no hard and fast rules for choosing a solution, *COMPROMISE* solutions usually have the best chance of being accepted by everyone. Each person must give a little to get a little.

<u>Leader</u>: Discuss each of the following rules with the group.

Rules for Brainstorming
1. **List as many solutions as you can.**
2. **Don't be critical. All ideas are allowed.**
3. **Be creative.**
4. **Begin by offering to change one of your own behaviors.**

<u>Leader</u>: Ask students to suggest some typical parent-teenager problems, and write them on the blackboard. Then select one of the problems and have the students generate as many solutions as possible. Remind them to try to come up with some solutions that parents would also find acceptable. Go through several problems with the group, and list the solutions under them on the blackboard. (Make sure there are some solutions that would appeal to parents.) *HIGHLIGHT* the solutions that are compromises. Leave the problems and solutions on the blackboard for a later exercise.

WORKBOOK

Ask students to turn to page 12.1. Have them answer questions #1 and #2.

III. CHOOSING A SOLUTION (15 min.)

Objectives
1. To present a systematic method for narrowing down the list of ideas that are generated during the brainstorming stage.
2. To practice evaluating solutions.

Next, we're going to learn how to choose one solution to try from the list of ideas that have been generated during the brainstorming stage. This can be difficult because *EVERYONE INVOLVED HAS TO AGREE* on the solution to the problem; otherwise it won't work. Remember that *COMPROMISE SOLUTIONS* usually have a better chance of being selected. The rule for this session is that compromise is the key to reaching mutual agreements.

┌─────────────┐
│ WORKBOOK │   Ask students to turn to page 12.2.
└─────────────┘

We're going to use the Problem-Solving Worksheet on page 12.2 to help us evaluate each of the possible solutions. This worksheet has been designed for teenagers and parents, although it could be used by anyone. Each solution that has been suggested during the brainstorming stage is given either a *PLUS OR A MINUS* by each person involved. This is a quick way to find out which ideas are acceptable to everyone.

At this stage, each person must state *WHY* he or she thinks a particular solution is good or bad. When you do this, it's important to be *POSITIVE*. Don't just turn down an idea because you don't like it. The goal is to find a solution that will resolve the problem.

Let's consider an example.

THE PROBLEM

Mom   "It bothers me when you leave your clothes all over your room. I'm embarrassed to invite my friends into the house because they might see the mess in there. I think we need to work on this problem. Let's begin by brainstorming some possible solutions and then we'll choose one to try out. I'll write them down. Let's take turns—you go first."

BRAINSTORMING

Teenager   *(Solution #1)* "We could hire a maid to clean up my room."

Mom   *(Solution #2)* "I could withhold your allowance until you cleaned your room."

Teenager   *(Solution #3)* "We could just shut the door to my room when we have company."

Mom   *(Solution #4)* "I could pay you an extra five dollars if you cleaned your room by Sunday night.

                    "OK, I think we have enough ideas. I'll read them one at a time and we'll take turns giving each of the possible solutions a plus or a minus."

EVALUATION

Mom	"The first solution is to hire a maid."

Teenager "That sounds good to me—then I wouldn't have to clean up my room! I give that idea a plus."

Mom "Hiring a maid would be great if I could afford it, but I really can't. I'm afraid I have to give that idea a minus unless we win the state lottery.

"The second solution is to withhold your allowance until your room is clean."

Teenager "That doesn't seem fair. If I forget to clean my room, I don't get any money at all. I'm going to give that idea a minus."

Mom "I think withholding your allowance would motivate you to keep your room clean, and you would still have a choice about whether or not you wanted to do it. I give that idea a plus.

"The third solution is to keep the door to your room closed."

Teenager "Shutting the door seems like a great idea. It's my room and I should get to do what I want in there. If I keep the door closed, the mess wouldn't bother you or your friends. I give that idea a plus."

Mom "Closing the door would keep other people from seeing what a mess your room is, but it wouldn't help you learn to be responsible for keeping your room clean. I give that idea a minus.

"The last solution is to pay you five dollars for cleaning your room by Sunday night."

Teenager "I like that idea. That way, I could earn some extra money, and you wouldn't have to nag me about my room anymore. I'm giving that solution a plus."

Mom "Paying you some extra money for cleaning your room seems like a good idea to me, too. You would learn to take care of your room, and it would be clean by Sunday night. That would be worth five dollars a week to me! I give that idea a plus.

"Since we both agree on this one, let's give it a try! Thanks for helping me work on the problem."

Team Activity

Leader: Ask students to form teams by pairing up.

The first step is for each of you to copy this parent-teenager problem [go to the blackboard and indicate which one] **and the proposed solutions onto page 12.2. Then one team member will play the part of the parent, and the other will play the part of the teenager as you *EVALUATE* each of the solutions. Use page 12.2 as your worksheet for this exercise. As you evaluate the solutions, keep in mind that each person must state *WHY* a particular solution is good or bad.**

Leader: When most of the teams have finished, ask team members to present some of their evaluations to the rest of the class.

Break (10 min.)

Let's take a *10-minute* break.

IV. IMPLEMENTATION AND CONTRACTING (15 min.)

Objective
1. To discuss how to write a contract that spells out the details of a solution.

Once you have come to an agreement about which solution to try, *ALL OF THE DETAILS* need to be spelled out in a *WRITTEN CONTRACT*. The contract is a formal record of the terms and conditions that you have negotiated. It establishes the *EXACT WORDING* of the agreement, which is very important if there are any questions or disputes about what was said. *BE SPECIFIC* when you write the contract so it's easy to evaluate whether each person is upholding his or her part of the agreement. Describe what should happen in language that is observable and behavioral—remember our discussions about baselining at the beginning of the course.

The contract should describe *WHAT EACH PERSON WILL DO* and *WHAT WILL HAPPEN* (the consequence) *IF EITHER PARTY FAILS TO UPHOLD THE AGREEMENT.* Even though people may have good intentions, they often fail to follow through on their promises. You can provide some additional incentive to honor the agreement by including a consequence.

The contract should also spell out the *PERIOD OF TIME* it is good for. This is particularly important because you may find that you want to change the agreement. However, you should stick to the agreement for the *ENTIRE PERIOD OF TIME* specified in the contract. Otherwise, the contract may not be taken seriously. It takes time to find out whether the agreement is going to work, so give it a try for at least a week. At the end of the trial period, review the agreement, and consider each person's suggestions regarding changes that would make the agreement work better.

INCLUDE REMINDERS to help you remember to make the changes that have been agreed upon. People often forget what they are supposed to do, so it's important to use cues or reminders.

Leader: Students may reject this last idea because they want to be treated like adults and feel that they don't need reminders (also, reminders may seem like nagging). Point out, however, that we all need prompts when we are trying to change well-established habits. Offer some examples of appropriate cues: (a) put the agreement on the refrigerator or in some other public place; and (b) post a note in the bedroom, on the mirror, or in some other place where it will be seen frequently. Brainstorm some other ideas with students.

| WORKBOOK |

Ask students to turn to page 12.3.

Leader: Review the contract on page 12.3 and discuss exactly how the details must be spelled out so that each person understands what he or she is expected to do. Have the group participate in making up a sample agreement.

V. PRACTICING PROBLEM SOLVING AND NEGOTIATION (35 min.)

Objective
1. To help students "put it all together" by having them work on a problem using all of the steps for problem solving and negotiation.

Team Activity

<u>Leader</u>: The goal here is to give all students an opportunity to work through an entire problem-solving sequence before they try to help their parents learn the steps for problem solving at home (this is part of their homework assignment for Sessions 13 and 14). While students are doing the following activity, spend some time with each team and give students constructive feedback.

WORKBOOK	Ask students to turn to pages 12.4 and 12.5.

<u>Leader</u>: Tell students to use the following steps for the team activity.

BLACKBOARD

> 1. Define the problem.
> 2. Brainstorm solutions.
> 3. Evaluate solutions.
> 4. Pick a solution (compromise).
> 5. Write a contract.

<u>Leader</u>:

1. Ask students to form "families" by having them pair up or get together in groups of three.

2. Have each "family" choose one of the problems listed on the blackboard that hasn't already been used in an exercise.

3. Start out by having one of the "families" role play a problem-solving interaction (using the Problem-Solving Worksheet on page 12.4) while the other "families" watch.

4. After *5 to 7 minutes*, have the "family members" change roles so that everyone has a chance to play a parental role. (This is important for developing an appreciation of the parent's perspective.)

5. Provide ongoing feedback to all "family members" regarding their communication and problem-solving performances. (Those playing the role of parents should also receive feedback.)

6. If sufficient progress has been made, have the "family members" write a contract (page 12.5) while the next "family" gets started.

7. Have another "family" role play a problem-solving interaction.

8. Continue until each "family" has participated in the exercise. All students should have had an opportunity to role play the part of the adolescent and the parent.

VI. HOMEWORK ASSIGNMENT (10 min.)

| WORKBOOK | Ask students to turn to the "For Adolescent Only Groups" homework assignment on page 12.6. |

1. **Your goal for this session is for you and your parents to complete the Issues Checklist. Write this on page 1.2. Your copy of the Issues Checklist is provided on pages 12.11 through 12.15. You will need to use the checklist during the next two sessions to help you decide which problems to work on.**

2. **I'm going to hand out some extra copies of the Issues Checklist. I want you to ask each of your parents or guardians to fill one out so you can bring it to the next two sessions. This will help you pick problems that your parents want to solve too.**

Leader: Hand out extra copies of the Issues Checklist. Give each student one or two copies depending on how many parents/guardians the student has living at home. Stress the importance of having the parent(s) fill out the Issues Checklist. If necessary, discuss any misgivings that the adolescents may have about asking their parents to fill it out.

3. **Complete the sample brainstorming and evaluation situations on pages 12.9 and 12.10.**

Leader: Briefly review pages 12.9 and 12.10, answering questions until you are satisfied that the students understand the assignment.

4. **Continue to monitor your daily mood by filling out your Mood Diary on page 1.1.**

5. **Remember to keep up your level of pleasant activities.**

6. Try to practice using the relaxation techniques, particularly in stressful situations.

   Are there any questions?

Success Activity

Let's do some of our homework right now. Fill out your Mood Diary for today.

Preview the Next Session

Next session, we'll devote all of our class time to practicing what we have learned about problem solving and negotiation.

VII.   QUIZ   (5 min.)

| WORKBOOK |

Ask students to take the quiz on brainstorming and evaluation on page 12.8.

<u>Leader</u>: After everyone has finished, read the answers out loud and have each student correct his or her own quiz.

SESSION 12 QUIZ
Negotiation and Problem Solving, Part 2

1. Which of the following are rules for brainstorming?

True	False		
(T)	F	a.	List as many solutions as you can.
T	(F)	b.	Each person should only offer one solution.
(T)	F	c.	Compromise is important.
T	(F)	d.	Stop after coming up with five solutions.
T	(F)	e.	Don't propose creative solutions.
(T)	F	f.	Offer to change one of your own behaviors.
(T)	F	g.	Don't be critical of other people's solutions.
T	(F)	h.	Evaluate each solution as soon as it is proposed.

   1 pt. each

2. Which of the following are rules for making a problem-solving contract?

True	False		
T	(F)	a.	It isn't necessary to write down a contract.
(T)	F	b.	The contract should describe what each person has agreed to do.
(T)	F	c.	The contract should indicate a point in time to evaluate the agreement to see if it's working as planned.
(T)	F	d.	The contract should spell out the period of time the contract is good for.

Continued on the next page

254

SESSION 12 QUIZ (continued)

<u>True</u>   <u>False</u>

  T   Ⓕ   e. If one person fails to uphold the terms of the agreement even *once*, then the contract is broken.

  T   Ⓕ   f. Once it's signed, the contract should be put away in a drawer; it should *not* be put up on display.

  Ⓣ   F   g. Contracts should include reminders to help each person keep his or her part of the agreement.

  T   Ⓕ   h. Contracts are only useful for solving problems in a family; they would *not* be useful for solving problems between friends.

SESSION 13A
Negotiation and Problem Solving, Part 3

Adolescent Only Version

Materials needed for this session:
1. Extra workbooks.
2. Copies of page 13.2.
3. Extra pens and pencils.
4. Refreshments for the break.
5. A kitchen timer.
6. Some blank audiotapes.

<u>Leader</u>: Write the steps for problem solving on the blackboard (see page 13.1 in the student workbook).

BLACKBOARD

AGENDA
I. HOMEWORK REVIEW (10 min.)
II. GUIDED PROBLEM SOLVING AND NEGOTIATION (70 min.)
Break (10 min.)
III. PRESENTING PROBLEM SOLVING TO PARENTS (20 min.)
IV. HOMEWORK ASSIGNMENT (10 min.)

I. HOMEWORK REVIEW (10 min.)

| WORKBOOK | Ask students to turn to pages 12.9 and 12.10.

<u>Leader</u>: Briefly review the answers for pages 12.9 and 12.10. Make sure that all students are given an opportunity to respond.

Check to make sure students are filling out the Mood Diary every day.

II. GUIDED PROBLEM SOLVING AND NEGOTIATION (70 min.)

Objective
1. To have students role play a complete problem-solving and negotiation session of mild to moderate intensity, using problems selected from the Issues Checklists completed by adolescents and their parents.

<u>Leader</u>: It will take *70 minutes* to complete this section: *10 minutes* to explain the process, and *60 minutes* for role playing. Use the following chart to determine how to divide up the *60 minutes* of role-playing time according to the number of students participating in the activity.

Number of Students		Each Student is Allocated
1	....	60 minutes
2	....	30 minutes
3	....	20 minutes
4	....	15 minutes
5	....	12 minutes
6	....	10 minutes
7	....	8 minutes
8	....	7 minutes

<u>Leader</u>: Stop for a *10-minute break* about two-thirds of the way through this activity. The exact timing of the break will depend on the duration of the your group's role plays—don't interrupt students in the middle of a problem-solving interaction to take the break.

Group Activity

<u>Leader</u>: The goal for this activity is to have each student participate in a problem-solving and negotiation practice session. Pairs of students will take turns participating in the exercise while the other students watch.

During the exercise, sit near the student who is role-playing the adolescent and guide the problem-solving interaction and provide prompts and praise. The following is the recommended seating arrangement:

(Group Leader)---> GL

(student role playing teenager)---> T   P <---(student role playing parent)

```
            X      +-------+      X
                   |       |
            X      | table |      X
                   |       |
(other students)   X       |      X
    --->           X       |      X
                   X       |      X
                   +-------+
              X        X
```

<u>Leader</u>: Briefly explain the following instructions for this exercise to the entire group.

Now that you have learned the steps involved in problem solving and negotiation, we're going to practice using them.

| WORKBOOK | Ask students to turn to pages 12.11 through 12.15.

The first thing you need to do is to go over the topics on the Issues Checklist, which is the questionnaire you filled out as part of your homework assignment last week; I hope you were able to get each of your parents to fill one out as well. You will need to *PICK ONE TOPIC* that both you and your parents agree is still a problem, but only a low-level or *MILD PROBLEM*. We will work up to dealing with the "hot" or troublesome topics later on.

Then, we will form a "family" by having one of you role play the part of the teenager who is presenting an issue and someone else role play the part of the parent. Each of you will take turns working on the problem you have selected from the checklist, using the steps for problem solving. To make things a little easier, we will use the Problem-Solving Worksheet that you have used before as a guide for the discussion; a copy of this is provided on page 13.2 in the workbook. We used this worksheet last week in class, so it should be very familiar to you.

<u>Leader</u>: Write the steps for problem solving on the blackboard, if you haven't done this already. It will save time if you do this before the beginning of the session. Mention that these steps are also provided on page 13.1. Briefly discuss each step (allow *1 minute* each).

BLACKBOARD

> Define the Problem
> 1. One person states the problem by describing what the other person is doing or saying that creates the problem.
> 2. The other person uses active listening (restates the problem).
> 3. The first person verifies the accuracy of the restatement of the problem.
>
> Brainstorm
> 1. List all possible solutions.
> 2. Be creative.
> 3. Don't be critical.
> 4. Compromise.
> 5. Think about changing your own behavior.

BLACKBOARD (continued)

> Choose a Solution
> 1. Each person evaluates the solutions and explains why each one is a "plus" or a "minus."
> 2. Fill out the Problem-Solving Worksheet.
> 3. Compromise.
>
> Write a Contract
> 1. Describe what each person will do, and what will happen if he or she fails to do it.
> 2. State how long the contract is good for.
> 3. Include reminders.
> 4. Sign the contract.

I want to make this practice session as easy as possible for you. I will sit next to you and offer assistance if you need it as you go through the steps for problem solving. Try to relax and have fun with this exercise, and don't worry about doing it perfectly the first time. Your approach will improve with practice—that's what this session is all about.

The goal for each you is to work through as much of one problem as possible in the time available. We will use this timer [hold it up] to keep track of how much time you have.

The first step is to come up with a good *DEFINITION* of the problem so that your discussion gets off to a good start. Then, you will spend some time *BRAINSTORMING* possible solutions, and *EVALUATING* at least some of them.

[If there are only a few students, add the following statement.] "If there is enough time, each of you can write and sign a contract that describes the details of the agreement you have negotiated during this practice session."

At the end of the exercise, I will give you some *FEEDBACK* about the problem-solving discussion. The feedback will involve pointing out the things you did well and indicating the areas that could use some improvement.

We will begin this exercise by asking one of you to volunteer to role play the part of the teenager and we will need another volunteer to role play the part of the parent. The rest of you will watch as they go through the practice session, and then I will ask two more of you to volunteer. We will repeat this process until everyone has had a chance to practice problem solving and has received some feedback.

Leader: The general instructions for the guided practice are as follows:

1. Ask for a volunteer to role play the part of him- or herself. It would be best to begin with someone who can provide a good role model for the other students. Try to pick a student who will do relatively well with this process. Ask for a second volunteer to role play the part of the teenager's parent.

2. Have the student who is playing him- or herself *SELECT AN ISSUE THAT IS ONLY MILDLY DISTRESSING* for the teenager and his or her parent(s). If the Issues Checklist is used, ask the student to pick a topic with an intensity rating of 1 or 2, but no higher. If the Issues Checklist has not been completed by the student and/or the parent(s), have the student scan the list and select an issue that is of mild intensity. It isn't necessary for the student to spend a lot of time trying to pick the "ideal" issue to solve; the goal for this session is not to solve a major problem, but to *PRACTICE* the necessary skills.

┌─────────────────┐
│ **WORKBOOK** │ Ask students to turn to page 13.2.
└─────────────────┘

3. Ask the "parent" to be the *SECRETARY*. Explain that it's the secretary's job to record the solutions and evaluations generated during the discussion on the Problem-Solving Worksheet on page 13.2.

4. Ask the "teenager" to *DEFINE* the problem using the rules discussed earlier. (The eight rules are: 1. start with positive; 2. be specific; 3. describe what the other person is doing; 4. no name-calling; 5. express your feelings; 6. admit your role; 7. don't accuse; and 8. be brief.) Make sure the definition is specific and behaviorally descriptive.

5. Have the "parent" respond to the problem statement with *ACTIVE LISTENING* (paraphrase, use feeling statements, etc.). Make sure this is done correctly. If necessary, acknowledge that this may feel awkward or artificial, but ask them to continue.

6. Have the "teenager" *VERIFY* whether the active-listening statements accurately reflect what he or she has said. If not, have both participants repeat the process of defining the problem and responding with active listening.

7. Next, have them go through the *PROBLEM-SOLVING STEPS* listed on the blackboard.

8. During the discussion, *PROVIDE ONGOING FEEDBACK*. Label and praise good performances out loud. If either person moves too quickly, is critical and evaluates solutions during brainstorming, etc., give immediate feedback by gently reminding that person about the relevant rule.

9. When approximately *3 minutes* of the allocated time remain (depending on the number of students), stop the discussion, and *PROVIDE MORE DETAILED FEEDBACK* to the students involved in the practice session.

10. Select two more students (or reverse the roles of the two students who just finished the practice session), and repeat the process.

11. Continue until all students have had an opportunity to role play a problem-solving discussion.

12. If there is enough time, have the students *WRITE A CONTRACT* by filling out the form on page 13.3. Another option is to ask some of the students who were having difficulties to *DO SOME ADDITIONAL PRACTICE*.

III. PRESENTING PROBLEM SOLVING TO PARENTS (20 min.)

Objective
1. To help students develop a positive approach for convincing their parents to learn problem-solving techniques and practice using them.

Now that you have had some practice using the steps for problem solving here in class, we are going to ask you to try to *SOLVE SOME SMALL PROBLEMS AT HOME, WITH YOUR PARENTS*. Of course, your parents probably don't know the steps for problem solving that we have discussed in class. So, your job will be to:

1. ***PRESENT THE IDEA* of doing some problem solving to your parents, in a positive way. The goal is to get them to agree to *PRACTICE AT LEAST TWICE*.**

2. ***BRIEFLY TEACH YOUR PARENTS THE STEPS* for effective problem solving. The worksheets and guidelines in your workbook will make this part of your job a little easier.**

How can you convince your parents to try problem solving? Let's think of some things you can do to make this easy for you, and to make it more likely that your parents will agree to help out.

a. **When would be a good *TIME* to bring this up? When would be a bad time?**

(Answer—Good Times: Ask parents to suggest a good time to get together to talk; make an appointment with parents to talk; when parents are relaxed, not during a fight; when both parents are around, so you can all agree on a convenient time for a meeting.)

(Answer—Bad Times: Right after parents get home from work, and they are tense; during a fight or argument; when other activities have already been planned, for example, guests are coming over for dinner; when parents are busy with household chores.)

WORKBOOK   Ask students to turn to page 13.5.

Leader: Have each student identify the two best times to present the problem-solving assignment to his or her parents. Ask students to write this down at the top of page 13.5.

b. **Where would be a good *PLACE* to bring this up? Where would be a bad place?**

(Answer—Good Places: At the dinner table, after supper; in the living room when both parents are there; at home.)

(Answer—Bad Places: In a store or other public place; in the car; in a crowd, or when other people are around.)

Leader: Have each student identify the two best places to present the problem-solving assignment to his or her parents. Ask students to write this down on page 13.5.

c. **What would be a good way to SAY it? What would be a bad
    way? (Hint: remember the communication skills discussed
    earlier?)**

*Answer—Good Ways to Say It: "Mom/Dad, remember the group
I've been going to? Well, there is some kind of homework
assignment for every session. This time I need to have you help
me, since the homework involves practicing with other people." or,
"I'm supposed to practice a certain way of solving problems that
I've learned in class. It's called negotiation. The practice involves
picking a problem that both the parents and the teenager want to
solve, and going through some steps to negotiate a solution. I've
got some forms from the class that will make it easy." or, "I would
really appreciate it if you could help me practice something that I
need to do for class."*

*Answer—Bad Ways to Say It: "Hey, you guys have to do this with
me! My group leader said you need to compromise on a problem
with me." or, "You've got to pick a problem that you're screwing
up on, and we've got to change what you're doing about it."*

**Try to emphasize that this is practice, and that your parents are helping you out
by practicing the problem-solving steps with you.**

Leader: Have students brainstorm some ways to ask their parents to practice problem solving
together. Have each student write down what he or she will say in the space provided at the
bottom of page 13.5.

d. **What are some problems that might come up? What are some possible
    solutions?**

Leader: Work with students to identify problems and possible solutions. Some students will
probably be extremely *pessimistic* (and perhaps even scared) about approaching their parents.
Try to convince them to at least give it a try. The following are some possible problems.

i. *Problem:* **Your parents are too busy.**
    Solution: **Use a calendar to make an appointment with your
    parents. Be willing to give up some activity of your own (for
    example, a favorite TV show, shopping, etc.) in order to
    schedule a meeting time.**

ii. *Problem:* You are so convinced that your parents will refuse to help that you won't ask them, or you ask in a way that turns them off.
Solution: Spend some time analyzing your thoughts using the C-A-B method. Are your beliefs about your parents irrational? Should you try to ask them, and give it your *best* try?

iii. *Problem:* Your parents refuse to help, even when you have tried your best to get them to cooperate.
Solution: Maybe there is someone else who would be willing to practice with you. Parents are the best choice, but if this doesn't work out, try asking your friends, brothers/sisters, minister etc.

iv. *Problem:* Your parents don't understand why it's important to learn about problem solving and negotiation.
Solution: Show your parents the pages in the workbook that deal with problem solving. Use these pages to explain how this approach can help you solve problems that are creating conflict without anyone getting angry. Emphasize that this will help you gain control over your mood.

<u>Leader</u>: Use brainstorming and evaluation skills (and forms, if necessary) to help identify problems and possible solutions. Stress the importance of doing this homework assignment.

Teaching Your Parents

Helping your parents learn how to solve problems will be a step-by-step process, just like it was for you. A summary of the teaching steps is provided at the bottom of page 13.5. Let's briefly review these steps.

1. Show your parents page 13.1 in your workbook. Go through the steps.

2. Show your parents how to use the Problem-Solving Worksheet on page 13.2 and the Agreement Contract on page 13.3.

3. Remember, this is supposed to be a practice session! It's OK to look at the list of steps, and to go slowly. It will take at least an hour to describe the approach to your parents and practice working on a problem.

IV. HOMEWORK ASSIGNMENT (10 min.)

```
┌─────────────┐
│ WORKBOOK    │
└─────────────┘
```
Ask students to turn to the "For Adolescent Only Groups" homework assignment on page 13.4.

1. Your goal for this session is to work on a problem with your parents. Write this on page 1.2.

2. Before you leave, you need to make a commitment to ask your parents to help you practice problem solving. Follow the notes you have written down on page 13.5 to guide your choice of the time and place to ask them, and use the dialogue you have written at the bottom of the page to present the idea to your parents. Once they have agreed to help you, set a time for a practice session.

3. Get together with your parents at the specified time and go through the teaching procedure at the bottom of page 13.5.

4. Practice working on the problem you selected in class, or choose another problem from the Issues Checklist. Go through the problem-solving steps listed on page 13.1 as you negotiate a solution. Use the Problem-Solving Worksheet on page 13.7 to take notes. Try to reach a solution and fill out the contract on page 13.8 if you can, but make sure you end the practice session within a reasonable length of time (60 to 90 minutes). You can always meet again to continue the practice session.

5. Once you have an agreement in writing, *PUT IT INTO PRACTICE.*

6. If any of you didn't fill out the Issues Checklist last session, please do so before the next session.

7. If problems develop or tempers flare up during the discussion at home, it may be a good idea to take a *TIME OUT*. A time out is a 10- to 15-minute break that allows everyone to calm down. Make sure that the discussion continues after the break is over.

8. Another useful technique for practicing problem solving and negotiation at home is to *AUDIOTAPE* the discussion so that I can give you some feedback and suggestions. If you are interested in doing this, there are some blank audiotapes available. I will be the only one who will listen to the tapes—*they will not be shared with the group.*

9. Continue to fill out your Mood Diary every day (page 1.1).

Are there any questions?

Preview the Next Session

Next session, we'll practice the steps for problem solving and negotiation again. This time, however, you will be asked to pick a topic that is a little more distressing than the one you worked on during this session. *IT'S IMPORTANT TO DO YOUR HOMEWORK SO THAT YOU CAN GET THE MOST OUT OF THE NEXT SESSION.*

Leader: There is no quiz this session.

SESSION 14A
Negotiation and Problem Solving, Part 4

Adolescent Only Version

Materials needed for this session:
1. Extra workbooks.
2. Copies of page 14.1.
3. Extra pens and pencils.
4. Refreshments for the break.
5. A kitchen timer.

BLACKBOARD

> **AGENDA**
> I. HOMEWORK REVIEW (45 min.)
> II. MORE PROBLEM SOLVING AND
> NEGOTIATION (60 min.)
> *Break (10 min.)*
> III. HOMEWORK ASSIGNMENT (5 min.)

I. HOMEWORK REVIEW (45 min.)

<u>Leader</u>: The goal in this section is to review the homework assignment, provide praise and constructive feedback, and problem solve any difficulties each student may have had with his or her family during the practice session at home.

WORKBOOK   Ask students to turn to pages 13.7 and 13.8.

<u>Leader</u>: Ask each student to describe how his or her parents responded to the idea of using problem-solving techniques to work on family issues. Students are likely to mention some difficulties they experienced in getting their parents to cooperate. Address these difficulties by having the other students *briefly* brainstorm some suggestions to help each student successfully complete a practice session with his or her parents.

Have the students who conducted a problem-solving session with their parents report on how it went. Other students can help brainstorm solutions to any problems each family may have had while problem solving or implementing the contract.

COLLECT THE AUDIOTAPES of the home practice sessions and, if possible, *MAKE PHOTOCOPIES* of the Problem-Solving Worksheet (page 13.7) and the Agreement Contract (page 13.8) each student's family generated.

Check to make sure that students are filling out the Mood Diary (page 1.1).

II. MORE PROBLEM SOLVING AND NEGOTIATION (60 min.)

Objective
1. To have students role play a complete problem-solving and negotiation session of moderate intensity, using problems selected from the Issues Checklist completed by the students and their parents.

<u>Leader</u>: Use the following chart to determine how to divide up the *60 minutes* of role-playing time according to the number of students participating in the activity.

Number of Students		Each Student Is Allocated
1	....	60 minutes
2	....	30 minutes
3	....	20 minutes
4	....	15 minutes
5	....	12 minutes
6	....	10 minutes
7	....	8 minutes
8	....	7 minutes

<u>Leader</u>: Stop for a *10-minute break* about two-thirds of the way through this activity. The exact timing of the break will depend on the duration of the role plays—don't interrupt students in the middle of a problem-solving interaction to take the break.

Group Activity

<u>Leader</u>: The goal for this activity is to give students additional practice using the steps for problem solving and negotiation.

This activity is very similar to the one you participated in last session. If you finished your homework assignment from the last session, you will be asked to pick another topic from the Issues Checklist to work on. This time, the issue can be one that's slightly more distressing than the one you selected last time. Try to find a topic with an intensity rating of 3 to 5, but no higher. Those of you who didn't finish your homework assignment can use your time in the activity to prepare to complete your assignment as homework for this session.

<u>Leader</u>: The general instructions for the guided practice are as follows:

1. Work with the students who completed their homework first.

2. Ask for a volunteer to role play the part of him- or herself. Have the student *SELECT AN ISSUE THAT IS SLIGHTLY MORE DISTRESSING* than the one he or she worked on last time. If the Issues Checklist is used, have the student pick a topic with an intensity rating of 3 to 5, but no higher.

WORKBOOK	Ask students to turn to page 14.1.

3. Ask the student who is role playing him- or herself to be the *SECRETARY*. It will be this student's responsibility to record the solutions and evaluations generated during the practice session on the Problem-Solving Worksheet on page 14.1; if an agreement is reached, it should be recorded on page 14.2.

4. Ask for a second volunteer to role play the part of the parent.

WORKBOOK   Ask students to turn to page 13.1.

5. Remind the students to follow the problem-solving steps listed on page 13.1 to guide their practice session.

6. Ask one student to *DEFINE* the problem using the established rules. Make sure the definition is specific and behaviorally descriptive. If the student who is role playing the part of the "teenager" defined the problem during the last practice session, have the "parent" define the problem this time, and vice versa.

7. Have the other student respond to the problem statement with *ACTIVE LISTENING* (paraphrase, use feeling statements, etc.). Make sure this is done correctly.

8. Ask the person who stated the problem to *VERIFY* whether the active-listening statements accurately reflect what he or she has said.

9. Next, have the "family" go through as many of the *PROBLEM-SOLVING STEPS* as possible.

10. During the discussion, *PROVIDE ONGOING FEEDBACK*. Label and praise good performances out loud. If either person moves too quickly, is critical, evaluates solutions during brainstorming, etc., give immediate feedback by gently reminding that person about the relevant rule on page 13.1.

11. When approximately *3 minutes* remain of the allocated time (depending on the number of students), stop the discussion and *PROVIDE MORE DETAILED FEEDBACK* to each of the students involved in the role-playing session.

12. Select two more students (or reverse the roles of the two students who just finished the practice session), and repeat the process.

13. Continue until all students have had an opportunity to role play a problem-solving discussion.

14. If there is enough time, ask the students to *WRITE A CONTRACT* using page 14.2. Another option is to have some of the students who were having difficulties *DO SOME ADDITIONAL PRACTICE*.

III. HOMEWORK ASSIGNMENT (5 min.)

| WORKBOOK | Ask students to turn to the "For Adolescent Only Groups" homework assignment on page 14.3.

1. **Your goal for this session is to work on another problem with your parents or to complete the one you started last time. Write this on page 1.2.**

2. **Select a time and place to ask your parents to participate in another problem-solving practice session, and write this down on page 14.3 in your workbook. Do this before you leave class!**

3. **Once they have agreed to help you, set a time and place for the practice session.**

4. **At the agreed upon time, get together with your parents and: a) if you didn't finish your assignment from the last session, go through the remaining steps until you reach an agreement, *or* b) if you finished your assignment, work on a problem of moderate intensity (it can be the problem you selected for the practice session in class today, or something else). If you need them, there is a Problem-Solving Worksheet on page 14.5 and an Agreement Contract on page 14.5.**

5. **You may want to audiotape your practice session so I can give you some feedback. If you are interested in doing this, there are some blank audiotapes available.**

6. **Once you have an agreement in writing, *PUT IT INTO PRACTICE*.**

7. **Continue to fill out your Mood Diary every day (page 1.1).**

Are there any questions?

Preview the Next Session

Next session, we'll discuss how to write a life plan that will help you overcome feelings of depression in the future.

<u>Leader</u>: There is no quiz for this session.

SESSION 15
Life Goals

Materials needed for this session:
1. Extra workbooks.
2. Extra pens and pencils.
3. Refreshments for the break.

BLACKBOARD

AGENDA
- I.   HOMEWORK REVIEW (15 min.)
- II.   LIFE PLAN (40 min.)
  Break (15 min.)
- III. OVERCOMING FEARS AND OBSTACLES (35 min.)
- IV. HOMEWORK ASSIGNMENT (10 min.)
- V.   QUIZ (5 min.)

I. HOMEWORK REVIEW (15 min.)

Before we move on, let's review the material we covered during the last two sessions. I'm going to ask some questions—please raise your hand if you think you know the answer.

Oral Review/Quiz

1. **Why are problem solving and negotiation important?**
    (Answer: They are essential skills for resolving disagreements and building friendships.)

2. **Name some of the basic rules for defining a problem.**
    (Answer: Start with something positive; be specific; describe what the other person is doing or saying; no name-calling; express your feelings; admit your contribution to the problem; don't accuse; be brief.)

3. **When you have finished problem solving, what kind of agreement do you make with the other person?**
    (Answer: A written contract.)

4. **What are the important parts of a contract?**
    (Answer: The contract should describe what each person will do and what will happen (the consequences) if either person fails to uphold the terms of the agreement; it's also necessary to establish the period of time the contract is good for, and to set a date for reviewing the contract.)

Review Student Progress/Record Forms

A. **Session Goal (page 1.2)**

1. **Were you successful at upholding the terms of your contract (page 13.3 and/or page 14.2/14.5)? What problems did you have? Did you revise your contract?**

B. Mood Monitoring (page 1.1)

   1. Are you recording your mood rating every day?

C. Problem Solving

   1. Did any of you practice defining a problem with your family or friends since the last session? How did the other person respond? Did it help the situation?

   2. Did anyone negotiate a solution to a problem? With whom? How did it work? What (if anything) went wrong?

<u>Leader</u>: Briefly address the difficulties mentioned by students in using problem-solving techniques, and brainstorm some ways to improve their approach.

D. Other Skills (optional)

   1. Did you practice using active listening? How did it work?

   2. Are you maintaining your level of pleasant activities?

   3. Are you practicing the Benson and Jacobsen relaxation techniques?

II. LIFE PLAN (40 min.)

Objectives

1. To distinguish between long-term and short-term goals.
2. To help each student determine his or her goals in specific areas of life.
3. To guide students as they formulate a set of long-term goals.

The Importance of Long-Term Goals

So far, we have been working on *SHORT-TERM GOALS* that describe the things we need to do on a *DAILY OR WEEKLY* basis. It's also important to have *LONG-TERM GOALS* because they give us *DIRECTION*. Long-term goals describe what we are striving for or the type of person we *EVENTUALLY* want to be. Short-term goals help us reach long-term goals by pointing out the *SMALL STEPS* we need to take to get there.

For example, if you wanted to become a guitar player in a professional rock-n-roll band, that would be a long-term goal. What would your short-term goal be if you want to reach that long-term goal?
(Answer: Practice the guitar every day for three or four hours.)

During the last several weeks, we've been learning how to reach short-term goals (for example, raising our level of pleasant activities week by week). In this session, we're going to talk about setting some long-term goals. It's important to know what your long-term goals are because they *POINT OUT NEW SHORT-TERM GOALS* that will help you take steps in the right direction.

1. For example, suppose you weigh 160 pounds and you would like to weigh 140 pounds. What is your long-term goal?
    (Answer: To weigh 140 pounds; to lose 20 lbs.)

2. What would be a good short-term goal?
    (Possible answer: Skip dessert every day; eat one-fourth less on every plate; allow a maximum of 1500 calories each day; exercise three times every week; lose two pounds per week; etc.)

3. What are the two important things to remember in making short-term goals?
    (Answer: Be SPECIFIC, and be REALISTIC—establish goals that are a slight improvement over baseline).

Setting Realistic Long-Term Goals

It's also important to be specific and realistic when we are setting long-term goals. Sometimes, however, it's difficult to know whether long-term goals are realistic. Because long-term goals focus on where you want to be in the future, they tend to assume a lot of improvement and change. Long-term goals can become *UNREALISTIC* when we expect changes that are *TOO BIG*.

For example, we could probably become concert pianists if we practiced eight hours a day for 200 years. The problem is that we won't live that long. Only those of us with exceptional talent can become concert pianists in one lifetime. This would be a realistic long-term goal for some people, but for most of us it isn't.

4. **If you are 5' 8" and large-boned, would it be a realistic long-term goal to weigh 110 lbs.?**
   (Answer: No, it would be unrealistic as well as unhealthy. A more realistic goal would be to weigh 135-145 lbs, for both girls and boys according to standard weight charts for 16- to 18-year-olds.)

The Life Plan Worksheet

> **WORKBOOK**   Ask students to turn to page 15.1.

There is a chart of *CATEGORIES* for goals on page 15.1. The first category is *FRIENDS*. Write the name of a potential friend in this box. Then think of the obstacles that might get in the way of making friends with this person, and write them in the second box. Leave the last set of boxes (Plans for Overcoming Obstacles) blank for right now.

1. **What are some possible obstacles?**
   (Answer: Not having an opportunity to see the person, not being able to talk to the person, etc.)

<u>Leader</u>: Guide the students as they continue through the remaining categories on the Life Plan Worksheet.

Team Activity

<u>Leader</u>: Time limit: *15-20 minutes.*

Form teams by pairing up. Then, review each other's list of life goals on page 15.1. Discuss your life goals with your partner. Help each other decide whether the goals are specific and realistic. What are some short-term goals that would help you reach your long-term goals? Review the potential obstacles too. Are they realistic? Are there other obstacles?

<u>Leader</u>: Tell students not to fill in the boxes for overcoming obstacles until after the break.

Break (15 min.)

Let's take a *15-minute* break. We deserve a longer break today!

III. OVERCOMING FEARS AND OBSTACLES (35 min.)

Objective
1. To discuss some of the fears that can hold students back from reaching goals, and to consider some ways to overcome them.

People are often afraid of the future. The reasons for this include:
1. **Fear of *CHANGE*. People become comfortable with the way things are. Even if the current situation isn't the greatest, people are often afraid that things might get worse.**
2. **Fear of the *UNKNOWN*. Uncertainty about what will happen in the future can be upsetting. For example, what kind of job will you have? Where will you live? Will you go to college? etc.**
3. **Fear of *FAILURE*. People your age often worry about things like not getting into college, flunking out of college, being unemployed, not living up to their parents' expectations, etc.**
4. **Fear of *DYING*. Thoughts about being killed in a car accident or just getting old can be very disturbing.**
5. **Fear of *CONFLICT* with parents or friends. Differences may arise over goals and expectations that create distance between you and significant others.**

These types of fears are perfectly natural, and they are experienced to some degree by virtually all adolescents and adults. However, if we don't control these fears, they can *HOLD US BACK* from reaching important individual goals. For example, fear of the unknown may keep you from applying to out-of-state colleges, or it may keep you from calling someone for a date, studying for an exam, or applying for a job.

One of the best ways to deal with your concerns is to plan for the future. This involves doing the following:
1. **Setting some long-term goals—we've already done this on page 15.1.**
2. **Identifying possible obstacles.**

3. Coming up with some ways to overcome those obstacles.

Overcoming Obstacles

Group Activity

Leader: Time limit: *25 minutes.*

Each of you listed several long-term goals on page 15.1. You also listed several things that could get in the way of reaching your goals. Now, we are going to try to find some ways to overcome those obstacles.

Leader: Help students come up with strategies for overcoming each of the obstacles they have listed on page 15.1. Encourage them to draw from the skills covered earlier in the course such as problem solving, assertiveness, and negotiation. Do as much of this exercise out loud, as a group, as time will allow. When most of the students have completed this exercise, ask them to share what they have written on their Life Plan Worksheets (i.e., read the goal, the possible obstacles, and the plan for overcoming the obstacles). Then ask the rest of the students to provide appropriate feedback and suggestions.

IV. HOMEWORK ASSIGNMENT (10 min.)

| WORKBOOK | Ask students to turn to the homework assignment on page 15.2. |

1. **Continue to monitor your daily mood using page 1.1.**

2. **Practice using the Benson and Jacobsen relaxation techniques, especially in stressful situations.**

3. **Begin recording your pleasant activities again. Use page 15.4 or continue where you left off on page 2.4.**

All of you are encouraged to begin recording pleasant activities again. The two main reasons for doing this are to keep in practice, and to get you into the habit of "reactivating" the skills you have learned when you need them. It's important for you to be able to do this after the course is over—to start using

specific skills again from time to time, when you are feeling down as well as just to keep in practice.

4.   Turn to your Session Goal Record on page 1.2 and write, "Monitor mood, practice relaxation, and record pleasant events."

Are there any questions?

Success Activity

Let's do some of our homework right now.
1.   Write down your mood score for today on page 1.1.
2.   Record the pleasant activities you have done today on page 15.4 or 2.4.

Preview the Next Session

The next session is our last class together. You have put a lot of effort into learning a whole new set of skills for taking control of your life and changing how you feel. Congratulations for staying with it! Next session, we'll learn how to maintain our gains and plan for the future.

V.   QUIZ   (5 min,)

WORKBOOK   Ask students to take the quiz on life goals on page 15.4.

Leader: After everyone has finished, read the answers out loud and have each student correct his or her own quiz.

Make sure to fill out a certificate of graduation for each student before the final session. A blank form that can be photocopied is provided in the appendices of this manual.

SESSION 15 QUIZ
Life Goals

1. How do short-term goals help you reach long-term goals?

   They help break long-term goals into reasonable steps

2. The following are some long-term goal statements. Write an "R" next to the goals that are realistic, and a "U" next to goals that are unrealistic.

   U   a. Bob's family is lower-middle income; they live in a small, but comfortable house. Bob has $200 saved up to buy a car. He has a part-time job, and he earns about $100 each month. Bob's goal is to buy a $5000 car by the beginning of summer next year, which is nine months away.

   R   b. Wendy is a good freshman athlete. She is on the cross country track team and competes in long-distance races. Wendy is one of the best runners in her school. At several recent track meets, she placed second and third. Wendy's goal is to win first place in her event by the end of her senior year.

   U   c. Mary's goal is to become a major rock star by the time she is twenty, and she wants to sell a million copies of her first album. She listens to a lot of records, and knows the lyrics to most of the songs by her favorite groups. She doesn't know anyone in the music business, and can't play any instruments.

   R   d. Jack likes to ski, and has been skiing since he was five years old. He gives lessons to beginning skiers on weekends. Jack's long-term goal is to become a designer of ski equipment. He has taken several drafting and engineering classes, and has done well in these classes. He has been accepted into a college that has a very good engineering program.

Continued on next page

3. Bill doesn't have as many friends as he'd like, so his goal is to make more friends. One of the major obstacles for Bill is that he lives far away from the people he'd like to be friends with, and it would be difficult to get together with them. The following are some possible solutions. Write a "G" next to the solutions that are good and a "B" next to the solutions that are bad.

B   a. Bill could ask his dad to let him use the car in the afternoon. This would mean that his dad would have to take a forty-minute bus ride to work.

G   b. Bill could take the bus to visit his friends.

G   c. Bill could make plans to meet his friends on weekends and arrange to use his dad's car when it's free.

B   d. Bill could spend most of his time with a kid in his neighborhood who is four years younger than he is.

1 pt. each

284

SESSION 16
Prevention, Planning, and Ending

Materials needed for this session:
1. Extra workbooks.
2. Extra pens and pencils.
3. Refreshments for the break.
4. A certificate of graduation for each student.

BLACKBOARD

AGENDA

     I.   HOMEWORK REVIEW (15 min.)
    II.   MOOD QUESTIONNAIRE (15 min.)
   III.   MAINTAINING GAINS (15 min.)
   IV.   EMERGENCY PLANNING (25 min.)
       Break (15 min.)
    V.   EARLY RECOGNITION (10 min.)
   VI.   SUMMARY (15 min.)
  VII.   ENDING THE COURSE (10 min.)

I.   HOMEWORK REVIEW (15 min.)

Let's begin by reviewing some of the material we covered during the last session. I'm going to ask some questions—please raise your hand if you think you know the answer.

Oral Review/Quiz

1. **How do short-term goals help us reach long-term goals?**
   (*Answer: They break down large changes into small steps.*)

2. **What are two important things to remember when making short-term goals?**
   (*Answer: Be SPECIFIC, and be REALISTIC—a slight improvement over baseline.*)

3. **Kelly is a freshman. She weighs about 115 pounds, and her doctor has told her this is about all she'll ever weigh. She is a good athlete, and participates in many sports. Her goal is to play football on the boys' team, and she wants to be a starting defensive guard by next year. The average weight of the defensive guards on the team is 195 pounds. Is this a realistic long-term goal for Kelly?**
   (*Answer: No, she doesn't weigh enough.*)

4. **What if Kelly wanted to play on the boys' baseball team? Size and weight are not as important in this sport. Is this a realistic goal for Kelly?**
   (*Answer: Yes, it's a realistic goal as long as she plays as well as the other members of the team—and assuming that the school is open-minded about mixed-sex sports teams.*)

Review Student Progress/Record Forms

A. Session Goals

1. Have you been monitoring your mood every day (page 1.1)?
2. Have you noticed any improvement in your mood?
3. Have you been practicing relaxation? Which version (Jacobsen or Benson) seems to work best for you?
4. Did you record your pleasant activities?
5. Are you keeping up your overall level of pleasant activities?

II. MOOD QUESTIONNAIRE (15 min.)

Objectives
1. To have each student fill out a Mood Questionnaire.
2. To compare the "Beginning of the Course" score with the "End of the Course" score.

| WORKBOOK | Ask students to turn to the "End of the Course" Mood Questionnaire in the Appendix. |

The first thing we're going to do today is fill out a Mood Questionnaire. I will be the only one reading your responses, so please answer honestly.

Leader: After everyone has finished, give instructions for scoring.

To score the questionnaire, add up all the numbers you have circled. If you have circled more than one number for a statement, add only the largest number to your score. You may notice that the numbers for your responses on four of the statements (#4, #8, #12, and #16) are listed in reverse order. This has been done on purpose, and your score will be correct if you simply add up the numbers you have circled.

After you have scored the questionnaire, _COMPARE_ your score from today with your score on the same questionnaire at the beginning of the course.

I hope that many of you notice a decrease in your scores. If you don't see any decrease, however, don't feel too discouraged. Some people experience a _DELAYED REACTION_ to the course, and their moods don't improve until several weeks later.

For those of you who don't see a decrease in your score, have you noticed any other positive changes? For example, do you see a trend in your Mood Diary; has your relationship with your parents improved; are you getting along better with your friends; are you doing better in school; etc.?

Leader: Collect the completed Mood Questionnaires from the students. Check the scoring and record the totals during the break. Return the questionnaires to the students after the break.

III. MAINTAINING GAINS (15 min.)

Objective
1. To help each student identify everyday problem areas and select skills to cope with them.

Each one of you has put a lot of work into practicing new skills and trying *NEW WAYS OF THINKING AND BEHAVING* in this course. I hope that you have found something that will help you gain control over your mood.

We all experience everyday hassles or problems from time to time. This is normal. However, these *SMALL THINGS CAN OCCASIONALLY OVERWHELM US* and make us feel depressed.

If steps are taken to *MAINTAIN THE GAINS* you have made, you can minimize the effects of these everyday hassles. Remember—it's easier to *PREVENT* problems than it is to get rid of them once they get started.

| WORKBOOK |

Ask students to turn to page 16.1.

Assign priorities to your problem areas using the worksheet on page 16.1. Which ones are most important for you to work on?

1. What are your major "everyday" problem areas? Don't include major catastrophes or major stressors. Just list *HASSLE* situations.
2. Describe some ways to cope with these everyday problems. Which *SKILLS* are most effective for dealing with these everyday issues? Are these skills ones that you can use every day? How about every week?
3. Decide how you can *REMIND* yourself to use these skills on a daily or weekly basis. What kind of reminders work best for you?

4. In order to prevent depression, try to *BUILD THESE TECHNIQUES INTO YOUR DAILY LIFE* so that you can deal with everyday hassles effectively.

<u>Leader</u>: Ask students which techniques work best for them in dealing with everyday hassles and problems.

IV. EMERGENCY PLANNING (25 min.)

Objectives
1. To have each student generate a list of major life events that may occur in the future.
2. To help each student consider how these events will affect his or her behavior, and then come up with a prevention plan.

Even if we practice our skills and try to maintain our gains, there will be times when we begin to feel depressed again. When this happens, it's important to remember that you can still do something to *HELP YOURSELF*.

The first step is to recognize the kinds of things that can cause or *"TRIGGER"* your depression. For most people, *MAJOR LIFE EVENTS* and life changes often lead to depression. These are more than just everyday hassles. Here are some examples:
1. *SOCIAL SEPARATIONS* **such as friends moving away, divorce, or the death of someone close to you.**
2. *HEALTH-RELATED PROBLEMS* **such as getting sick or injured.**
3. *NEW RESPONSIBILITIES AND ADJUSTMENTS* **such as a new job or transferring to a different school.**
4. *WORK-RELATED ISSUES* **such as stress from a job or too much work.**
5. *FINANCIAL CRISES* **such as not having enough money to pay the bills or losing your job.**
6. *MAJOR EVENTS HAPPENING TO SOMEONE CLOSE TO YOU* **such as a good friend moving away, or someone you enjoy working with getting fired.**

Life changes don't necessarily have to be negative to cause distress and/or depression. For example, moving, getting married, and graduating from high school can affect your mood. Even *POSITIVE CHANGES* can feel like a major upheaval in your life.

289

> | WORKBOOK | Ask students to turn to page 16.2.

What are the *MAJOR LIFE EVENTS* that might affect you in the near future? Some events are predictable (for example, graduation), but others may occur without warning (for example, someone stealing your car). Try to list some of the events that are relatively predictable. Which ones contribute to your depression?

Leader: Ask each student to list potential triggers for his or her depression in the first column on page 16.2. Solicit examples and write them on the blackboard. Are there some triggers that several students have in common? Ask students how they can learn to recognize trigger events early. Are there ways to avoid the major life events that are unpredictable? Stress that early recognition of depressive symptoms is critical.

Now that you know what your triggers are, you are ready to anticipate and plan for them. The next step is to think about how each trigger will *AFFECT YOUR BEHAVIOR*. For example, how will you act toward your family and friends?

Leader: Ask students to fill out the middle column on page 16.2.

Now look at the last column on page 16.2. In this column, develop a *PREVENTION PLAN* for each of the major life events you listed in the left-hand column. How can you keep from getting depressed, given the major life events you expect in the near future? Write your plans for preventing depression in the right-hand column.

Team Activity

Leader: If there is enough time before the break, have students form teams by pairing up or getting together in groups of three. Ask them to give their teammate suggestions about how to deal with the stressful events they are anticipating. Circulate among the groups, offering comments and making suggestions regarding the skills they have learned in class that might be useful. After each student has had a chance to discuss his or her major life events, bring the whole class back together to share ideas.

Break (15 min.)

Let's take a *15-minute* break.

V.   EARLY RECOGNITION (10 min.)

Objective

1.   To describe the symptoms of depression and to emphasize the importance of having students continue to monitor their moods.

As we mentioned earlier, preventing depression is far easier and less painful than treating depression when it has become much more severe. In addition to your Prevention Plan, it is also important to *RECOGNIZE SYMPTOMS AND SIGNS OF DEPRESSION EARLY*.

WORKBOOK   Ask students to turn to page 16.3.

Clinical depression has *SYMPTOMS*, just like a common cold or the flu. For example, some of the symptoms of the flu are a fever, aching muscles, headache, and loss of appetite. The symptoms of clinical depression are listed on page 16.3.

Review these symptoms carefully. If you have only one or two of them, it may not be clinical depression. But if you have several of these symptoms at the same time, and they are present for a minimum of one to two weeks, then it may be clinical depression.

In order to help prevent depression, you should *REVIEW THESE SYMPTOMS* every week or so. Do you have any of them? How long have you had them? Do you feel sad?

If you think you may be just a little bit depressed or sad, work on maintaining your gains (see page 16.1). If you are very depressed, either work on your Prevention Plan (page 16.2) or see your doctor or counselor.

Don't wait for the depression to go away on its own. Sometimes this happens, but it's better to *TAKE ACTIVE STEPS* to make it go away faster.

Here are some other ways to keep track of your depression and mood:
1. Fill out the Mood Questionnaire (once a week, once a month).
2. Use your Mood Diary (page 1.1).

Leader: Ask students to identify at least one way they will keep track of their moods over time. How will they remind themselves to do this?

VI. SUMMARY (15 min.)

Objective
1. To have students summarize their progress and evaluate the effectiveness of increasing pleasant activities and controlling thinking.

Since this is the last session, it's a good time to think about the changes you have made and all the things you have learned.

Here are some of the topics we have covered:
1. Relaxation techniques.
2. Increasing pleasant activities.
3. Changing negative thinking.
4. Friendly skills, improving relationships.
5. Active listening and self-disclosures (communication).
6. Negotiation and problem solving.
7. Making a life plan.

Which skills and/or techniques were most important for you?

Leader: Lead a brief discussion.

Remember the idea that your personality is a three-part system? Where have you noticed the most improvements?

BLACKBOARD

Actions
Thoughts
Feelings

Which skills do you need to continue to work on?

<u>Leader</u>: Have students discuss which areas they need to practice more.

VII.   ENDING THE COURSE (10 min.)

Closing Remarks

<u>Leader</u>: It's important to tailor the message you give here to the group of students. The specific words you use are less important than the process itself. The issues to think about are: Do the students have a sense of hope and optimism? Are their goals specific and realistic? Have they had a chance to share their feelings about the class experience? Is there a sense of closure?

Beginnings and endings are important times. Among other things, they provide an opportunity to plan and reflect.

We have formed a cohesive, supportive group, and each of us has come to depend on the group and its regular meetings in some way. Perhaps you should expect somewhat of a let-down as the course ends, and therefore it's important to develop a plan for dealing with that. For instance, you might want to increase your rate of pleasant activities during the coming week and, in particular, include some extra social activities.

<u>Leader</u>: Close with remarks about having enjoyed the group, being proud of the progress everyone has made, etc. Allow some time for others to make remarks, if they wish, and come to a sense of closure.

Use the remaining time for group socializing, making brief personal contacts with each adolescent. Give each student a certificate of graduation.

SECTION III
Parent + Adolescent Sessions

The modified versions of Sessions 12, 13, and 14 in this section should be used when parents participate in the program. Parents attend separate course sessions that are held once a week, on one of the same nights as the adolescent sessions (a *Leader's Manual for Parent Groups* and a *Parent Workbook* are available from the publisher for these course sessions).

The adolescent and parent groups are brought together for Sessions 13 and 14. During these sessions, each family practices the skills for communication, problem solving, and negotiation that they have learned earlier in the course. Some changes also have been made in Session 12 in preparation for these joint sessions.

SESSION 12
Negotiation and Problem Solving, Part 2

Adolescent + Parent Version

Materials needed for this session:
1. Extra workbooks.
2. Extra pens and pencils.
3. Refreshments for the break.

BLACKBOARD

AGENDA
    I. HOMEWORK REVIEW (15 min.)
    II. BRAINSTORMING (15 min.)
    III. CHOOSING A SOLUTION (15 min.)
    Break (10 min.)
    IV. IMPLEMENTING AND CONTRACTING (15 min.)
    V. PRACTICING PROBLEM SOLVING AND NEGOTIATION (35 min.)
    VI. HOMEWORK ASSIGNMENT (10 min.)
    VII. QUIZ (5 min.)

RULE: Compromise is the key to reaching mutual agreements.

I.   HOMEWORK REVIEW (15 min.)

Let's begin by reviewing some of the concepts that were discussed during the last session. I'm going to ask some questions—please raise your hand if you think you know the answer.

Oral Review/Quiz

1.   **What are the four steps for assertive-imagery practice?**
     (Answer: Make a mental photograph of the situation; convert the photograph into a movie; state your feelings in the movie; imagine the other person's reaction.)

2.   **Why is it important to learn problem-solving and negotiation skills?**
     (Answer: These are essential skills for resolving complaints and preventing minor conflicts from becoming serious. They help to maintain friendships and harmony.)

3.   **What are the two basic rules for successful problem solving?**
     (Answer: The person with a complaint has the right to be heard; listening to the complaint doesn't mean that you agree or disagree.)

4.   **What are the rules for defining a problem?**
     (Answer: Begin with something positive; be specific; describe what the other person is saying or doing; no name-calling; express your feeling; admit your contribution; don't accuse; be brief.)

Review Student Progress/Record Forms

A. **Session Goal (page 1.2)**

   1.   **Did you identify one or more problems that you would like to work on?**
   2.   **Did you record the problems on page 11.6, and practice defining them using the eight rules?**

298

B. **Mood Monitoring** (page 1.1)

1. **Are you remembering to record your mood rating every day?**
2. **Have you noticed any improvement in your mood?**

C. **Active Listening** (optional)

1. **Did you have any opportunities to practice active listening? How did it work?**
2. **Have you tried using active-listening skills in situations where someone was communicating a negative feeling?**

D. **Pleasant Activities** (optional)

1. **Did you meet your goal for pleasant activities (page 4.6)?**

E. **Relaxation Techniques** (optional)

1. **Did you use the relaxation techniques?**

II. BRAINSTORMING (15 min.)

Objectives
1. To discuss the rationale and rules for brainstorming.
2. To practice brainstorming by having students generate solutions to some typical parent-teenager problems.

During the last session, we discussed the importance of problem-solving and negotiation skills. We learned how to *DEFINE PROBLEMS* and how to respond with *ACTIVE LISTENING SKILLS* when someone else states a problem. In this session, we're going to learn *NEGOTIATION SKILLS* that will help us resolve issues by working with the other person to reach a mutual agreement.

After the problem has been *DEFINED* so that everyone understands what it is, the next step is to come up with a variety of *DIFFERENT SOLUTIONS* to the problem. At this stage, it's important to be creative and nonjudgmental. Don't be too hasty. Remember, none of the solutions to these problems has worked so far. The more ideas that everyone generates, the better. We call this approach *BRAINSTORMING*.

While there are no hard and fast rules for choosing a solution, *COMPROMISE* solutions usually have the best chance of being accepted by everyone. Each person must give a little to get a little.

<u>Leader</u>: Discuss each of the following rules with the group.

Rules for Brainstorming
1. **List as many solutions as you can.**
2. **Don't be critical. All ideas are allowed.**
3. **Be creative.**
4. **Begin by offering to change one of your own behaviors.**

<u>Leader</u>: Ask students to suggest some typical parent-teenager problems, and write them on the blackboard. Then select one of the problems and have the students generate as many solutions as possible. Remind them to try to come up with some solutions that parents would also find acceptable. Go through several problems with the group, and list the solutions on the blackboard. (Make sure there are some solutions that would appeal to parents.) *HIGHLIGHT* the solutions that are compromises. Leave the problems and solutions on the blackboard for a later exercise.

WORKBOOK

Ask students to answer questions #1 and #2 on page 12.1.

III. CHOOSING A SOLUTION (15 min.)

Objectives
1. To present a systematic method for narrowing down the list of ideas that are generated during the brainstorming stage.
2. To practice evaluating solutions.

Next, we're going to learn how to choose one solution to try from the list of ideas that have been generated during the brainstorming stage. This can be difficult because *EVERYONE INVOLVED HAS TO AGREE* on the solution to the problem; otherwise it won't work. Remember that *COMPROMISE SOLUTIONS* usually have a better chance of being selected. The rule for this session is that compromise is the key to mutual agreements.

WORKBOOK

Ask students to turn to page 12.2.

We're going to use the Problem-Solving Worksheet on page 12.2 to help us evaluate each of the possible solutions. This worksheet has been designed for teenagers and parents, although it could be used by anyone. Each solution that has been suggested during the brainstorming stage is given either a *PLUS OR A MINUS* by each person involved. This is a quick way to find out which ideas are acceptable to everyone.

At this stage, each person must state *WHY* he or she thinks a particular solution is good or bad. When you do this, it's important to be *POSITIVE*. Don't just turn down an idea because you don't like it. The goal is to find a solution that will resolve the problem.

Let's consider an example.

THE PROBLEM

Mom

"It bothers me when you leave your clothes all over your room. I'm embarrassed to invite my friends into the house because they might see the mess in there. I think we need to work on this problem. Let's begin by brainstorming some possible solutions and then we'll choose one to try out. I'll write them down. Let's take turns—you go first."

BRAINSTORMING

Teenager

(Solution #1) "We could hire a maid to clean up my room."

Mom

(Solution #2) "I could withhold your allowance until you cleaned your room."

Teenager

(Solution #3) "We could just shut the door to my room when we have company."

Mom

(Solution #4) "I could pay you an extra five dollars if you cleaned your room by Sunday night.

"OK, I think we have enough ideas. I'll read them one at a time and we'll take turns giving each of the possible solutions a plus or a minus."

EVALUATION

Mom   "The first solution is to hire a maid."

Teenager   "That sounds good to me—then I wouldn't have to clean up my room! I give that idea a plus."

Mom   "Hiring a maid would be great if I could afford it, but I really can't. I'm afraid I have to give that idea a minus unless we win the state lottery.

"The second solution is to withhold your allowance until your room is clean."

Teenager   "That doesn't seem fair. If I forget to clean my room, I don't get any money at all. I'm going to give that idea a minus."

Mom   "I think withholding your allowance would motivate you to keep your room clean, and you would still have a choice about whether or not you wanted to do it. I give that idea a plus.

"The third solution is to keep the door to your room closed."

Teenager   "Shutting the door seems like a great idea. It's my room and I should get to do what I want in there. If I keep the door closed, the mess wouldn't bother you or your friends. I give that idea a plus."

Mom   "Closing the door would keep other people from seeing what a mess your room is, but it wouldn't help you learn to be responsible for keeping your room clean. I give that idea a minus.

"The last solution is to pay you five dollars for cleaning your room by Sunday night."

Teenager   "I like that idea. That way, I could earn some extra money, and you wouldn't have to nag me about my room anymore. I'm giving that solution a plus."

| Mom | "Paying you some extra money for cleaning your room seems like a good idea to me, too. You would learn to take care of your room, and it would be clean by Sunday night. That would be worth five dollars a week to me! I give that idea a plus. |
| | "Since we both agree on this one, let's give it a try! Thanks for helping me work on the problem." |

Team Activity

<u>Leader</u>: Ask students to form teams by pairing up.

The first step is for each of you to copy this parent-teenager problem [go to the blackboard and indicate which one] **and the proposed solutions onto page 12.2. Then one team member will play the part of the parent, and the other will play the part of the teenager as you *EVALUATE* each of the solutions. Use page 12.2 as your worksheet for this exercise. As you evaluate the solutions, keep in mind that each person must state *WHY* a particular solution is good or bad.**

<u>Leader</u>: When most of the teams have finished, ask team members to present some of their evaluations to the rest of the class.

Break (10 min.)

Let's take a *10-minute* break.

IV. IMPLEMENTATION AND CONTRACTING (15 min.)

Objective

1. To discuss how to write a contract that spells out the details of a solution.

Once you have come to an agreement about which solution to try, *ALL OF THE DETAILS* need to be spelled out in a *WRITTEN CONTRACT*. The contract is a formal record of the terms and conditions that you have negotiated. It establishes the *EXACT WORDING* of the agreement, which is very important if there are any questions or disputes about what was said. *BE SPECIFIC* when you write the contract so it's easy to evaluate whether each person is upholding his or her part of the agreement. Describe what should happen in language that is observable and behavioral—remember our discussions about baselining at the beginning of the course.

The contract should describe *WHAT EACH PERSON WILL DO* and *WHAT WILL HAPPEN* (the consequence) *IF EITHER PARTY FAILS TO UPHOLD THE AGREEMENT.* Even though people may have good intentions, they often fail to follow through on their promises. You can provide some additional incentive to honor the agreement by including a consequence.

The contract should also spell out the *PERIOD OF TIME* it is good for. This is particularly important because you may find that you want to change the agreement. However, you should stick to the agreement for the *ENTIRE PERIOD OF TIME* specified in the contract. Otherwise, the contract may not be taken seriously. It takes time to find out whether the agreement is going to work, so give it a try for at least a week. At the end of the trial period, review the agreement, and consider each person's suggestions regarding changes that would make the agreement work better.

INCLUDE REMINDERS to help you remember to make the changes that have been agreed upon. People often forget what they are supposed to do, so it's important to use cues or reminders.

Leader: Students may reject this last idea because they want to be treated like adults and feel that they don't need reminders (also, reminders may seem like nagging). Point out, however, that we all need prompts when we are trying to change well-established habits. Offer some examples of appropriate cues: (a) put the agreement on the refrigerator or in some other public place; and (b) post a note in the bedroom, on the mirror, or in some other place where it will be seen frequently. Brainstorm some other ideas with students.

WORKBOOK

Ask students to turn to page 12.3.

Leader: Review the contract on page 12.3 and discuss exactly how the details must be spelled out so that each person understands what he or she is expected to do. Have the group participate in making up a sample agreement.

V. PRACTICING PROBLEM SOLVING AND NEGOTIATION (35 min.)

Objective
1. To help students "put it all together" by having them work on a problem using all of the steps for problem solving and negotiation.

Team Activity

Leader: The goal here is to give all students an opportunity to work through an entire problem-solving sequence before they attempt to do this with their parents (either at home, or during joint parent-student Sessions 13 and 14). While students are doing the following activity, spend some time with each team and give students constructive feedback.

> WORKBOOK   Ask students to turn to pages 12.4 and 12.5.

Leader: Tell students to use the following steps for the team activity.

BLACKBOARD

> 1. Define the problem.
> 2. Brainstorm solutions.
> 3. Evaluate solutions.
> 4. Pick a solution (compromise).
> 5. Write a contract.

Leader:
1. Ask students to form "families" by having them pair up or get together in groups of three.

2. Have each "family" choose one of the problems listed on the blackboard that hasn't already been used in an exercise.

3. Start out by having one of the "families" role play a problem-solving interaction (using the Problem-Solving Worksheet on page 12.4) while the other "families" watch.

4. After *5 to 7 minutes*, have the "family members" change roles so that everyone has a chance to play a parental role. (This is important for developing an appreciation of the parent's perspective.)

5. Provide ongoing feedback to all "family members" regarding their communication and problem-solving performances. (Those playing the role of parents should also receive feedback.)

6. If sufficient progress has been made, have the "family members" write a contract (page 12.5) while the next "family" gets started.

7. Have another "family" role play a problem-solving interaction.

8. Continue until each "family" has participated in the exercise. All students should have had an opportunity to role play the part of the adolescent and the parent.

VI. HOMEWORK ASSIGNMENT (10 min.)

> WORKBOOK   Ask students to turn to the "For Adolescent + Parent Groups" homework assignment on page 12.7.

1. **Your goal for this session is to complete the Issues Checklist on pages 12.11 through 12.15. Write this on page 1.2. You will need to use the checklist during the next two sessions to help you decide which problems to work on.**

2. **Complete the sample brainstorming and evaluation situations on pages 12.9 and 12.10.**

Leader: Briefly review pages 12.9 and 12.10, answering questions until you are satisfied that the students understand the assignment.

3. **Continue to monitor your daily mood by filling out your Mood Diary on page 1.1.**

4. **Remember to keep up your level of pleasant activities.**

5. **Try to practice using the relaxation techniques, particularly in stressful situations.**

Are there any questions?

Success Activity

Let's do some of our homework right now. Fill out your Mood Diary for today.

Preview the Next Session

Next session, we'll devote all of our class time to practicing what we have learned about problem solving and negotiation.

Leader: Remind the adolescents that their parents will be joining them in class for the next two sessions. Stress the importance of everyone attending. Have all students agree to attend the next two sessions. If necessary, briefly discuss any misgivings that the adolescents may have about the joint sessions.

VII.   QUIZ (5 min.)

WORKBOOK   Ask students to take the quiz on brainstorming and evaluation on page 12.8.

Leader: After everyone has finished, read the answers out loud and have each student correct his or her own quiz.

NOTE ABOUT PARENT-ADOLESCENT SESSIONS

Leader: The next two sessions are the joint parent-adolescent sessions (when parent groups are being conducted). Teen and parent group leaders should meet before Session 13 and rank-order the families according to their suspected ability to perform the problem-solving role plays. Start the role plays with the most accomplished families. Call the family at the top of the list to obtain their consent to go first in the Session 13 role plays.

SESSION 12 QUIZ
Negotiation and Problem Solving, Part 2

---

1. Which of the following are rules for brainstorming?

True	False		
(T)	F	a.	List as many solutions as you can.
T	(F)	b.	Each person should only offer one solution.
(T)	F	c.	Compromise is important.
T	(F)	d.	Stop after coming up with five solutions.
T	(F)	e.	Don't propose creative solutions.
(T)	F	f.	Offer to change one of your own behaviors.
(T)	F	g.	Don't be critical of other people's solutions.
T	(F)	h.	Evaluate each solution as soon as it is proposed.

   1 pt. each

2. Which of the following are rules for making a problem-solving contract?

True	False		
T	(F)	a.	It isn't necessary to write down a contract.
(T)	F	b.	The contract should describe what each person has agreed to do.
(T)	F	c.	The contract should indicate a point in time to evaluate the agreement to see if it's working as planned.
(T)	F	d.	The contract should spell out the period of time the contract is good for.

   1 pt. each

Continued on the next page

True	False	
T	(F)	e. If one person fails to uphold the terms of the agreement even *once*, then the contract is broken.
T	(F)	f. Once it's signed, the contract should be put away in a drawer; it should *not* be put up on display.
(T)	F	g. Contracts should include reminders to help each person keep his or her part of the agreement.
T	(F)	h. Contracts are only useful for solving problems in a family; they would *not* be useful for solving problems between friends.

SESSION 13
Joint Parent-Adolescent
Problem-Solving Session, Part 1

Adolescent + Parent Version

Materials needed for this session:
1. Extra workbooks.
2. Copies of page 13.2.
3. Extra pens and pencils.
4. Refreshments for the break.
5. A kitchen timer.
6. Some blank audiotapes.
7. Extra copies of the Issues Checklist.

<u>Leader</u>: Write the steps for problem solving on the blackboard (see page 13.1 in the *Student Workbook*).

BLACKBOARD

AGENDA
    I.   HOMEWORK REVIEW (10 min.)
    II.   GUIDED PROBLEM SOLVING AND
        NEGOTIATION (90 min.)
        Break (10 min.)
    III. HOMEWORK ASSIGNMENT (10 min.)

I. HOMEWORK REVIEW (10 min.)

| WORKBOOK | Ask students to turn to pages 12.9 and 12.10.

Student Group Leader. Briefly review the answers for pages 12.9 and 12.10, eliciting answers from adolescents and parents. Make sure that both adolescents and parents are given an opportunity to respond.

Parent Group Leader. Review the written contract that parents completed on *Parent Workbook* page 6.6.

Check to make sure students are filling out the Mood Diary every day.

II. GUIDED PROBLEM SOLVING AND NEGOTIATION (90 min.)

Objective

1.   To have parents and adolescents jointly participate in a problem-solving and negotiation session of mild to moderate intensity.

<u>Leader</u>: It will take *90 minutes* to complete this section: *10 minutes* to explain the process, and *80 minutes* for role playing. Use the following chart to determine how to divide up the *80 minutes* of role-playing time according to the number of families participating in the activity.

Number of Families		Each Family is Allocated
1	....	80 minutes
2	....	40 minutes
3	....	26 minutes
4	....	20 minutes
5	....	16 minutes
6	....	13 minutes
7	....	11 minutes
8	....	10 minutes

Leader: Stop for a *10-minute break* about halfway through this activity. The exact timing of the break will depend on the duration of the role plays—don't interrupt a family in the middle of a problem-solving interaction to take the break.

Family Activity

Leader: The goal for this activity is to have parents and adolescents practice problem solving and negotiation as a family. Each family will take turns participating in the exercise while the other families watch.

During the exercise, both the Student Group Leader and the Parent Group Leader should sit near their respective trainees so they can guide the problem-solving interaction and provide prompts and praise. The following is the recommended seating arrangement:

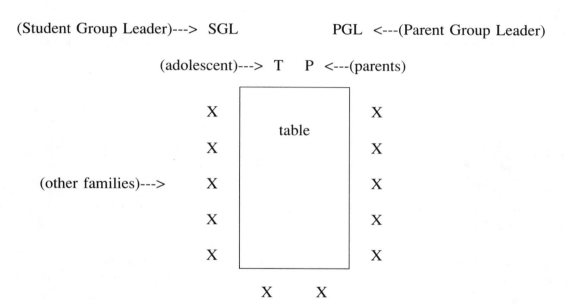

Leader: Briefly explain the following instructions for this exercise to the entire group.

Now that you have learned the steps involved in problem solving and negotiation, we're going to have each family practice them.

| WORKBOOK | Ask students to turn to pages 12.11 through 12.15. Ask parents to turn to pages 6.7 through 6.11. |

The first thing you need to do is to go over the topics on the Issues Checklist, which is the questionnaire you filled out as part of your homework assignment last week. Each family will need to *PICK ONE TOPIC* that the parents and the adolescent agree is still a problem, but only a low-level or *MILD PROBLEM*. We will work up to dealing with the "hot" or troublesome topics later on.

Then, each family will take turns working on the problem they have selected from the checklist, using the steps for problem solving. To make things a little easier, we will use the Problem-Solving Worksheet that you have used before as a guide for the discussion; a copy of this is provided on page 13.2 in the workbook. We used this worksheet last week in class, so it should be very familiar to you.

Leader: Write the steps for problem solving on the blackboard, if you haven't done this already. It will save time if you do this before the beginning of the session. Mention that these steps are also provided on page 13.1 in the *Student Workbook*. Briefly discuss each step (allow *1 minute* each).

BLACKBOARD

Define the Problem
1. One person states the problem by describing what the other person is doing or saying that creates the problem.
2. The other person uses active listening (restates the problem).
3. The first person verifies the accuracy of the restatement of the problem.

Brainstorm
1. List all possible solutions.
2. Be creative.
3. Don't be critical.
4. Compromise.
5. Think about changing your own behavior.

BLACKBOARD (continued)

> Choose a Solution
> 1. Each person evaluates the solutions and explains why each one is a "plus" or a "minus."
> 2. Fill out the Problem-Solving Worksheet.
> 3. Compromise.
>
> Write a Contract
> 1. Describe what each person will do, and what will happen if he or she fails to do it.
> 2. State how long the contract is good for.
> 3. Include reminders.
> 4. Sign the contract.

We want to make this practice session as easy as possible for you. Your group leaders will sit next to you while you go through the steps for problem solving, so they will be there to offer assistance if you need it. Try to relax and have fun with this exercise, and don't worry about doing it perfectly the first time. Your approach will improve with practice—that's what this session is all about.

The goal for each family is to work through as much of one problem as possible in the time available. We will use this timer [hold it up] to keep track of how much time each family has.

The first step is to come up with a good *DEFINITION* of the problem so that your discussion gets off to a good start. Then, you will spend some time *BRAINSTORMING* possible solutions, and *EVALUATING* at least some of them. The problem-solving steps that are not completed here will become your homework assignment. You should finish working through the remaining steps before the next session.

[If there are only a few families, add the following statement.] **"If there is enough time, each family can write and sign a contract that describes the details of the agreement that has been negotiated."**

At the end of the exercise, the group leaders will give each family some *FEEDBACK* about the problem-solving discussion. They will point out the things you did well, and they will also suggest areas that could use some improvement.

We will begin this exercise by asking one family to volunteer to go first while the other families watch. Then we will ask another family to volunteer. We will repeat this process until every family has had an opportunity to practice problem solving and has received some feedback.

Leader: The general instructions for the guided practice are as follows:

1. Ask one family to volunteer to go first. It would be best to begin with a family that will provide a good role model for the other families to follow.

2. Have the family *SELECT AN ISSUE THAT IS ONLY MILDLY DISTRESSING* for the parents and the adolescent. If the Issues Checklist is used, have them pick a topic with an intensity rating of 1 or 2, but no higher. If the Issues Checklist has not been completed by the parents and/or the adolescent, have them scan the list and select an issue that is of mild intensity. Tell them not to spend a lot of time trying to pick the "ideal" issue to solve; the goal for this session is not to solve a major problem, but to *PRACTICE* the necessary skills.

WORKBOOK	Ask students to turn to page 13.2.

3. Ask one family member to be the *SECRETARY*. Explain that it's the secretary's job to record all of the solutions and evaluations suggested by family members on the Problem-Solving Worksheet on page 13.2. Consider asking the family member who seems to be the least cooperative to be the secretary so that person will be actively involved in the process. Have all of the families who are watching also write down the solutions that are generated on a Problem-Solving Worksheet (pass out some extra copies); this will encourage them to pay attention to what is going on (which can sometimes be a problem for the families who are watching).

4. Have one family member *DEFINE* the problem using the rules discussed earlier. (The eight rules are: 1. start with positive; 2. be specific; 3. describe what the other person is doing; 4. no name-calling; 5. express your feelings; 6. admit your role; 7. don't accuse; and 8. be brief.) Make sure the definition is specific and behaviorally descriptive.

5. Ask the other members of the family to respond to the problem statement with ACTIVE LISTENING (paraphrase, use feeling statements, etc.). Make sure each person does this correctly. If necessary, acknowledge that this may feel awkward or artificial, but ask them to continue.

6. Have the person who stated the problem *VERIFY* whether the active-listening statements accurately reflect what he or she has said. If not, ask the family to repeat the process of defining the problem and responding with active listening.

7. Next, have the family go through the *PROBLEM-SOLVING STEPS* listed on the blackboard.

8. During the discussion, the Student Group Leader and the Parent Group Leader should *PROVIDE ONGOING FEEDBACK.* Make sure the group leaders label and praise good performances out loud. If a family member moves too quickly, is critical, evaluates solutions during brainstorming, etc., the group leaders should give immediate feedback by gently reminding that person about the relevant rule.

9. When approximately *5 minutes* of the allocated time remain (depending on the number of families), stop the discussion, and have the group leaders *PROVIDE MORE DETAILED FEEDBACK* to their respective trainees.

10. Select another family (or ask for volunteers), and repeat the process.

11. Continue until all families have had an opportunity to role play a problem-solving discussion.

12. If there is enough time, have the families *WRITE A CONTRACT* by filling out the form on page 13.3. Another option is to ask some of the families who were having difficulties to *DO SOME ADDITIONAL PRACTICE.*

III. HOMEWORK ASSIGNMENT (10 min.)

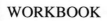

WORKBOOK
Ask students to turn to the "For Adolescent + Parent Groups" homework assignment on page 13.6. Parents should turn to the corresponding homework assignment in their workbooks.

1. Continue the discussion you have started in this session until you have completed all of the steps for problem solving and negotiation listed on the blackboard. These steps are also provided on page 13.1 in the workbook. Use the Problem-Solving Worksheet on page 13.2 to take notes. Before you leave, each family should try to come to a consensus about when to continue the discussion. If you can find a time that is convenient for everyone involved, write it down on page 13.6. Each person also needs to make a verbal commitment to participate in the problem-solving session. The goal is to agree on a solution and *WRITE A CONTRACT* using the form on page 13.3. Write this as your goal on page 1.2.

2. Once you have an agreement in writing, *PUT IT INTO PRACTICE.*

3. If any of you haven't filled out the Issues Checklist yet, please do so before the next session. Some extra copies of the checklist are available if you need them.

4. If problems develop or tempers flare during the discussion at home, it may be a good idea to take a *TIME OUT*. A time out is a 10- to 15-minute break that allows everyone to calm down. Make sure that the discussion continues after the break is over.

5. Another useful technique for practicing problem solving and negotiation at home is to *AUDIOTAPE* the discussion so that a group leader can give you some feedback and suggestions. If you are interested in doing this, there are some blank audiotapes available. Only the group leaders will listen to the tapes—*they will not be shared with the group.*

6. Students should continue to fill out the Mood Diary every day (page 1.1).

Are there any questions?

Preview the Next Session

Next session, we'll practice the steps for problem solving and negotiation again. This time, however, you will be asked to pick a topic that is a little more distressing than the one you worked on during this session. *IT'S IMPORTANT TO DO YOUR HOMEWORK SO THAT YOU CAN GET THE MOST OUT OF THE NEXT SESSION.*

<u>Leader</u>: There is no quiz this session. Have all family members agree to meet again for Session 14.

SESSION 14
Joint Parent-Adolescent
Problem-Solving Session, Part 2

Adolescent + Parent Version

Materials needed for this session:
1. Extra workbooks.
2. Copies of page 14.1.
3. Extra pens and pencils.
4. Refreshments for the break.
5. A kitchen timer.

<u>Leader</u>: Write the steps for problem solving on the blackboard (see page 13.1 in the *Student Workbook*).

BLACKBOARD

AGENDA
    I.   HOMEWORK REVIEW (40 min.)
    II. MORE PROBLEM SOLVING AND
        NEGOTIATION (65 min.)
        Break (10 min.)
    III. HOMEWORK ASSIGNMENT (5 min.)

I.   HOMEWORK REVIEW (40 min.)

Group Leaders. The goal for this section is to review the homework assignment, provide praise and constructive feedback, and problem solve any difficulties each family may have had during the practice session at home.

> WORKBOOK

Ask students to turn to pages 13.2 and 13.3.

Leader: Ask each family whether they held a meeting to continue the discussion they started in Session 13. Have them briefly describe their problem-solving interactions, their agreements, and the contracts they prepared (page 13.3). Ask them whether they were able to put the agreement into practice and whether it seems to be alleviating the problem. Make sure that the parents *and* the adolescent contribute to the discussion. If the family found it difficult to problem solve or to put the agreement into practice, the other families can help by brainstorming solutions.

COLLECT THE AUDIOTAPES of the home practice sessions and, if possible, *MAKE PHOTOCOPIES* of the Problem-Solving Worksheet (page 13.2) and the Agreement Contract (page 13.3) generated by each family.

Check to make sure students are filling out the Mood Diary (page 1.1).

II.   MORE PROBLEM SOLVING AND NEGOTIATION (65 min.)

Objective
1.   To have parents and adolescents jointly participate in a family problem-solving and negotiation session of moderate intensity.

Leader: Use the following chart to determine how to divide up the *65 minutes* of role-playing time according to the number of families participating in the activity.

Number of Families		Each Family Is Allocated
1	....	65 minutes
2	....	32 minutes
3	....	21 minutes
4	....	16 minutes
5	....	13 minutes
6	....	10 minutes
7	....	9 minutes
8	....	8 minutes

<u>Leader</u>: Stop for a *10-minute break* about halfway through this activity. The exact timing of the break will depend on the duration of the role plays—don't interrupt a family in the middle of a problem-solving interaction to take the break.

Family Activity

<u>Leader</u>: The goal for this activity is to give families additional practice using the steps for problem solving and negotiation. Families who completed the homework assignment from the last session can select a new problem from their Issues Checklist that is slightly more stressful than the one they worked on before. Begin with these families first. The families who didn't complete the homework assignment will use the time in this activity to finish the previous discussion and write a contract. Remind the families to use the problem-solving steps listed on the blackboard and on page 13.1. Then, briefly describe the exercise.

This activity is very similar to the one you participated in last session. If you finished your homework assignment from the last session, you will be asked to pick another topic from the Issues Checklist to work on. This time, the issue can be one that's slightly more distressing than the one you selected last time. Try to find a topic with an intensity rating of 3 to 5, but no higher. Those of you who didn't finish your homework assignment will use your time in the activity to come to an agreement and write a contract.

<u>Leader</u>: The general instructions for the guided practice are as follows.

1. Ask one family to volunteer to go first. Make sure it is a family who has completed the homework assignment from the last session.

2. Have them *SELECT AN ISSUE THAT IS SLIGHTLY MORE DISTRESSING* than the one they worked on last time. If the Issues Checklist is used, have them pick a topic with an intensity rating of 3 to 5, but no higher.

```
┌─────────────┐
│  WORKBOOK   │    Ask students to turn to page 14.1.
└─────────────┘
```

3. Ask one family member to be the *SECRETARY* (select someone other than the person who was secretary in Session 13). Have that person list all of the solutions and evaluations suggested by the family on the Problem-Solving Worksheet on page 14.1. Pass out some extra copies of page 14.1, and have the families who are watching also write down the solutions and evaluations.

4. Ask one family member to *DEFINE* the problem using the established rules. Make sure the definition is specific and behaviorally descriptive. If the adolescent defined the problem in Session 13, have the parents define the problem this time, and vice versa.

5. Have the other members of the family respond to the problem statement with *ACTIVE LISTENING* (paraphrase, use feeling statements, etc.). Make sure each person does this correctly.

6. Have the person who stated the problem *VERIFY* whether the active-listening statements accurately reflect what he or she has said.

7. Next, ask the family to go through as many of the *PROBLEM-SOLVING STEPS* as possible.

8. During the discussion, the Student Group Leader and the Parent Group Leader should *PROVIDE ONGOING FEEDBACK*. Make sure the group leaders label and praise good performances out loud. If a family member moves too quickly, is critical, evaluates solutions during brainstorming, etc., the group leaders should give immediate feedback by gently reminding that person about the relevant rule.

9. When approximately *5 minutes* remain of the allocated time (depending on the number of families), stop the discussion and have the group leaders *PROVIDE MORE DETAILED FEEDBACK* to their respective trainees.

10. Select another family (or ask for volunteers), and repeat the process.

11. Continue until all families have had an opportunity to role play a problem-solving discussion.

12.   If there is enough time, ask the families to *WRITE A CONTRACT* using page 14.2. Another option is to have the parents and adolescents *REVERSE ROLES* and repeat the process.

III. HOMEWORK ASSIGNMENT (5 min.)

WORKBOOK

Ask students to turn to the "For Adolescent + Parent Groups" homework assignment on page 14.4. Parents should turn to the corresponding homework assignment in their workbooks.

1.   **Try to stick with the agreement you have written down in your contract until the renegotiation date you have specified. Write this as your goal on page 1.2. On the renegotiation date, each family should meet again and decide whether to continue the current agreement or change it. Each of you will be asked to report on how the agreement is working out at the next session.**

2.   **Students should continue to fill out the Mood Diary every day (page 1.1).**

Are there any questions?

Preview the Next Session

Next session, we'll discuss how to write a life plan that will help you overcome feelings of depression in the future.

Leader: There is no quiz for this session.

APPENDICES

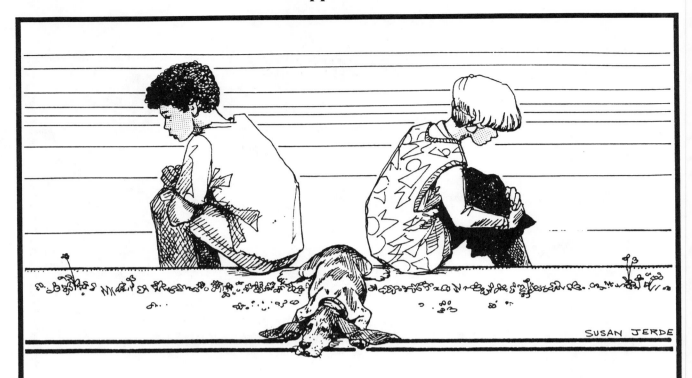

TEENS GET DEPRESSED TOO

Do you know a teenager who is sad or unhappy and bothered by:

- Low self-esteem or guilt
- Difficulty concentrating
- Loss of interest or pleasure
- Trouble sleeping

- Irritability
- Crying spells
- Loss of energy
- Loss of appetite

We can help you feel happier and better about yourself.
Oregon Research Institute and Oregon Health Sciences University
offer free small-group treatment for teenagers
(aged 14-18) who feel down or depressed.*

CALL 345-6505 (Eugene) OR 279-8476 (Portland)

*This treatment is being offered as part of an experimental study, and not all teenagers may qualify. Treatment is free for teenagers who qualify on the basis of an intake interview.

 Oregon Health Sciences University

Appendix 2

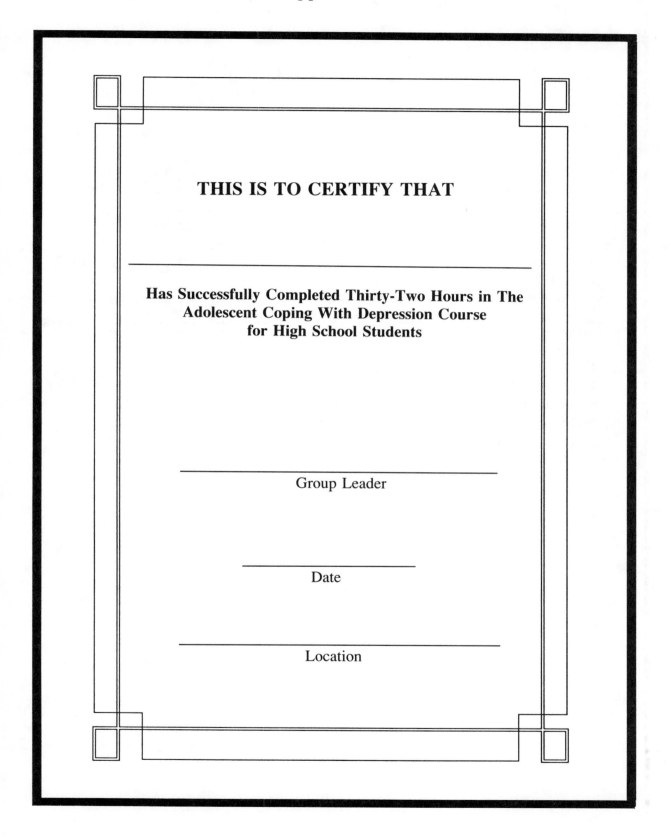

THIS IS TO CERTIFY THAT

_____

**Has Successfully Completed Thirty-Two Hours in The
Adolescent Coping With Depression Course
for High School Students**

_____

Group Leader

_____

Date

_____

Location

Appendix 3

Directions for Scoring the
Pleasant Events Schedule

The students should fill out the Pleasant Events Schedule—Adolescent Version during the intake interview (or sometime before they come to the first session). This information will be used for the baseline study of pleasant activities in Session 2, and it is therefore important to score the completed schedules in advance.

The schedule contains 320 items, and the purpose of "scoring" it is to help each student select 20 pleasant activities to work on. A computerized scoring program has been developed to make this easier, but it is also possible to generate a list of pleasant activities for each student by hand. The procedure involves reviewing the *PLEASURE* ratings assigned to each item and picking out the ones with the highest ratings first (i.e., "2"), then those with the next highest rating, until 30 or 40 pleasant activities have been identified for that individual. Instead of typing a list of activities for each student, it may be easier to simply put a checkmark next to the items on the schedule with the highest ratings. During Session 2, the students use the criteria provided on workbook page 2.5 to select 20 activities from the 30 or 40 that have been identified.

REFERENCES

Achenbach, T.M. The child behavior profile: I. Boys aged 6-11. *Journal of Consulting and Clinical Psychology*, 1978, **46**, 478-488.

Alexander, J.F. Defensive and supportive communications in normal and deviant families. *Journal of Consulting and Clinical Psychology*, 1973, **40**, 223-231.

Alexander, J.F., Barton, C., Schiavo, R.S., and Parsons, B.V. Systems-behavioral intervention with families of delinquents: Therapist characteristics, family behavior, and outcome. *Journal of Consulting and Clinical Psychology*, 1976, **44**, 656-664.

Alloy, L.B., and Abramson, L.Y. Judgment of contingency in depressed and non-depressed students: Sadder but wiser? *Journal of Experimental Psychology*, 1979, **108**, 441-485.

American Psychological Association. Ethical principles of psychologists. *American Psychologist*, 1981, 633-638.

Andrews, J.A., and Lewinsohn, P.M. *The prevalence of suicide attempts and the co-morbidity of suicide attempts with other psychiatric disorders.* Paper presented at the annual meeting of the American Psychological Association, New Orleans, (August) 1989.

Antonuccio, D.O., Akins, W.T., Chatham, P.M., Monagin, J.A., Tearnan, B.H., and Ziegler, B.L. An exploratory study: The psychoeducational treatment of drug-refractory unipolar depression. *Journal of Behavior Therapy and Experimental Psychiatry*, 1983, **15**, 309-313.

Bandura, A. (Ed.) *Social learning theory.* Englewood Cliffs, New Jersey: Prentice-Hall, 1977.

Bandura, A. Self-referent thought: A developmental analysis of self-efficacy. In J.H. Flavell and L. Ross (Eds.), *Social cognitive development: Frontiers and possible futures.* New York: Cambridge University Press, 1981.

Beck, A.T., Hollon, S.D., Young, J.E., Bedrosian, R.C., and Budenz, D. Treatment of depression with cognitive therapy and amitriptyline. *Archives of General Psychiatry*, 1985, **42**, 142-148.

References

Beck, A.T., Kovacs, M., and Weissman, A. Assessment of suicidal intention: The Scale for Suicidal Ideation. *Journal of Consulting and Clinical Psychology*, 1979, **47**, 343-352.

Beck, R.W., Morris, J.B., and Beck, A.T. The cross-validation of the Suicidal Intent Scale. *Psychological Reports*, 1974, **34**, 445-446.

Beck, A.T., Rush, A.J., Shaw, B.F., and Emery, G. *Cognitive therapy of depression: A treatment manual.* New York: Guilford Press, 1979.

Beck, A.T., Ward, C.H., Mendelson, M., Mock, J., and Erbaugh, J. An inventory for measuring depression. *Archives of General Psychiatry*, 1961, **4**, 561-571.

Bellack, A.S., Hersen, M., and Himmelhoch, J. Social skills training compared with pharmacotherapy and psychotherapy in the treatment of unipolar depression. *American Journal of Psychiatry*, 1981, **138**(12), 1562-1567.

Biglan, A., Hops, H., and Sherman, L. Coercive family processes and maternal depression. In R. DeV. Peters and R.J. McMahon (Eds.), *Social learning and system approaches to marriage and the family* (pp. 72-103). New York: Brunner/Mazel, 1988.

Blau, S. Guide to the use of psychotropic medications in children and adolescents. *Journal of Clinical Psychiatry*, 1978, **39**, 766-772.

Blechman, E.A., McEnroe, M.J., Carella, E.T., and Audette, D.P. Childhood competence and depression. *Journal of Abnormal Psychology*, 1986, **95**(3), 223-227.

Brown, R.A., and Lewinsohn, P.M. *Participant workbook for the Coping with Depression Course.* Eugene, Oregon: Castalia Publishing Company, 1984a.

Brown, R.A., and Lewinsohn, P.M. A psychoeducational approach to the treatment of depression: Comparison of group, individual, and minimal contact procedures. *Journal of Consulting and Clinical Psychology*, 1984b, **52**, 774-783.

Burns, D.D. *Feeling good: The new mood therapy.* New York: William Morrow Co., 1980.

Butler, L., Miezitis, S., Friedman, R., and Cole, E. The effect of two school-based intervention programs on depressive symptoms in pre-adolescents. *American Educational Research Journal*, 1980, **17**, 111-119.

Carlson, G.A. and Garber, J. Developmental issues in the classification of depression in children. In M. Rutter, C. Izard, and P. Read (Eds.), *Depression in young people: Developmental and clinical perspectives* (pp. 399-434). New York: Guilford Press, 1986.

Carver, C.S., and Scheier, M.F. An information-processing perspective on self-management. In P. Karoly and F.H. Kanfer (Eds.), *Self-management and behavior change: From theory to practice.* New York: Pergamon Press, 1982.

Chambers, W.J., Puig-Antich, J., Hirsch, M., Paez, P., Ambrosini, P.J., Tabrizi, M.A., and Davies, M. The assessment of affective disorders in children and adolescents by semi-structured interview: Test-retest reliability of the K-SADS-P. *Archives of General Psychiatry*, 1985, **42**, 696-702.

Chiles, J.A., Miller, M.L., and Cox, G.B. Depression in an adolescent delinquent population. *Archives of General Psychiatry*, 1980, **37**, 1179-1184.

Clarke, G.N. *A psychoeducational approach to the treatment of depressed adolescents.* University of Oregon, unpublished doctoral dissertation, 1985.

Clarke, G.N., Hops, H., Lewinsohn, P.M., and Andrews, J.A. *Cognitive-behavioral group treatment of adolescent depression: Prediction of outcome.* Unpublished manuscript, 1990.

Clarke, G.N., and Lewinsohn, P.M. *Leader manual for the Adolescent Coping with Depression Course.* Unpublished manuscript, Oregon Research Institute, 1986.

Clarke, G.N., and Lewinsohn, P.M. The Coping with Depression Course: A group psychoeducational intervention for unipolar depression. *Behavior Change*, 1989, **6**, 54-69.

References

Clarke, G.N., Lewinsohn, P.M., and Hops, H. *Leader's manual for adolescent groups: Adolescent Coping with Depression Course.* Eugene, Oregon: Castalia Publishing Company, 1990.

Clarke, G.N., Lewinsohn, P.M., Hops, H., and Andrews, J. *Cognitive-behavioral group treatment of adolescent depression: Prediction of outcome.* Reno, Nevada: Paper presented at the annual meeting of the Western Psychological Association, 1989.

Cole, T.L., Kelley, M.L., and Carey, M.P. The adolescent activities checklist: Reliability, standardization data, and factorial validity. *Journal of Abnormal Child Psychology,* 1988, **16**(5), 475-484.

Costello, E.J., Edelbrock, C.S., and Costello, A.J. Validity of the NIMH Diagnostic Interview Schedule for Children: A comparison between psychiatric and pediatric referrals. *Journal of Abnormal Child Psychology,* 1985, **13**, 579-595.

Coyne, J.C., Kessler, R.C., Tal, M., Turnbull, J., Wortman, C.B., and Greden, J.F. Living with a depressed person. *Journal of Consulting and Clinical Psychology,* 1987, **55**(3), 347-352.

DeRubeis, R.J., and Hollon, S.D. Behavioral treatment of affective disorders. In L. Michelson, M. Hersen, and S. Turner (Eds.), *Future perspectives in behavior therapy.* New York: Plenum, 1981.

Elkin, I., Parloff, M.B., Hadley, S.W., and Autry, J.H. NIMH Treatment of Depression Collaborative Research Project: Background and research plan. *Archives of General Psychiatry,* 1985, **42**, 305-316.

Ellis, A., and Harper, R.A. *A guide to rational living.* Hollywood, California: Wilshire Book, 1961.

Endicott, J., and Spitzer, R.L. A diagnostic interview: The Schedule for Affective Disorders and Schizophrenia. *Archives of General Psychiatry,* 1978, **35**, 837-844.

Frame, C., Matson, J.L., Sonis, W.A., Falkov, M.J. and Kazdin, A.E. Behavioral treatment of depression in a prepubertal child. *Journal of Behavior Therapy and Experimental Psychiatry,* 1982, **13**, 239-243.

Frank, J.D. Therapeutic components of psychotherapy: A 25-year progress report of research. *Journal of Nervous and Mental Disease*, 1974, **159**, 325-342.

Friedman, R.C., Hurt, S.W., Clarkin, J.F., Corn, R. and Aronoff, M.S. Symptoms of depression among adolescents and young adults. *Journal of Affective Disorders*, 1983, **5**, 37-43.

Forgatch, M.S., and Patterson, G.R. *Parents and adolescents living together, part 2: Family problem solving.* Eugene, Oregon: Castalia Publishing Company, 1989.

Goldklang, D.S. Research workshop on prevention of depression with recommendations for future research. *Journal of Primary Prevention*, 1989, **10**, 41-49.

Gonzales, L.R., Lewinsohn, P.M., and Clarke, G.N. Longitudinal follow-up of unipolar depressives: An investigation of predictors of relapse. *Journal of Consulting and Clinical Psychology*, 1985, **33**(4), 461-469.

Gottman, J., Notarius, C., Gonso, J., and Markman, H. *A couple's guide to communication.* Champaign, Illinois: Research Press, 1976.

Heiby, E.M. A Self-reinforcement questionnaire. *Behavior Research and Therapy*, 1983, **20**, 397-401.

Herjanich, B., and Reich, W. Development of a structured psychiatric interview for children: Agreement between child and parent on individual symptoms. *Journal of Abnormal Child Psychology*, 1982, **10**, 307-324.

Hirschfeld, R.M., and Cross, C.K. Epidemiology of affective disorders. *Archives of General Psychiatry*, 1982, **39**, 35-46.

Hoberman, H.M., and Lewinsohn, P.M. The behavioral treatment of depression. In E.E. Beckman and W.R. Leber (Eds.), *Handbook of depression: Treatment, assessment, and research* (pp 39-81). Homewood, Illinois: Dorsey Press, 1985.

Hoberman, H.M., Lewinsohn, P.M., and Tilson, M. Group treatment of depression: Individual predictors of outcome. *Journal of Consulting and Clinical Psychology*, 1988, **56**, 393-398.

References

Hollon, S.D. Clinical innovations in the treatment of depression: A commentary. *Advances in Behavior Research and Therapy*, 1984, **6**, 141-151.

Hollon, S.D., and Beck, A.T. Cognitive and cognitive behavioural therapies. In S.L. Garfield and A.E. Bergin (Eds.), *Handbook of psychotherapy and behaviour change* (pp. 443-482). New York: Wiley, 1987.

Hollon, S.D., Evans, M.D., and DeRubeis, R.J. Causal mediation of change in treatment for depression: Discriminating between nonspecificity and noncausality. *Psychological Bulletin*, 1987, **102**(1), 139-149.

Holmes, T.H., and Rahe, R.H. The social readjustment rating scale. *Psychosomatic Medicine*, 1967, **11**, 213-218.

Hops, H., Biglan, A., Sherman, L., Arthur, J., Friedman, L., and Osteen, V. Home observations of family interactions of depressed women. *Journal of Consulting and Clinical Psychology*, 1987, **55**(3), 341-346.

Hops, H., Lewinsohn, P.M., Andrews, J.A., and Roberts, R.E. Psychosocial correlates of depressive symptomatology among high school students. *Journal of Clinical Child Psychology*, in press.

Jacobsen, E. *Progressive relaxation*. Chicago: University of Chicago Press, 1929.

Kandel, D.B., and Davies, M. Epidemiology of depressive mood in adolescents: An empirical study. *Archives of General Psychiatry*, 1982, **39**, 1205-1212.

Kashani, J.H., Holcomb, W.R. and Orvaschel, H. Depression and depressive symptoms in preschool children from the general population. *American Journal of Psychiatry*, 1986, **143**, 1138-1143.

Kaslow, N.J., and Rehm, L.P. Conceptualization, assessment, and treatment of depression in children. In P.H. Bornstein and A.E. Kazdin (Eds.), *Handbook of clinical behavior therapy with children* (pp. 599-657). Homewood, Illinois: Dorsey Press, 1985.

Kazdin, A.E. Assessment of childhood depression: Current issues and strategies. *Behavioral Assessment*. 1987, **9**(3), 291-320.

Kazdin, A.E. Childhood Depression. In E.J. Mash and L.G. Terdal (Eds.), *Behavioral assessment of childhood disorders* (pp. 157-195). New York: Guilford Press, 1988.

Kazdin, A.E., Colbus, D., and Rodgers, A. Assessment of depression and diagnosis of depressive disorder among psychiatrically disturbed children. *Journal of Abnormal Child Psychology*, 1986, **14**, 499-515.

Kazdin, A.E., Sherick, R.B., Esveldt-Dawson, K., and Rancurello, M.D. Nonverbal behavior and childhood depression. *Journal of the American Academy of Child Psychiatry*, 1985, **24**, 303-309.

Keller, M.B., Shapiro, R.W., Lavori, P.W., and Wolfe, N. Relapse in major depressive disorder: Analysis of the life table. *Archives of General Psychiatry*, 1982, **39**, 911-915.

Klein, D.F., Gittelman, R., Quitkin, F., and Rifkin, A. *Diagnosis and drug treatment of psychiatric disorders.* Baltimore, Maryland: Williams and Wilkins, 1980.

Klerman, G.L. and Weissman, M.M. Increasing rates of depression. *Journal of the American Medical Association*, 1989, **261**, 2229-2235.

Kramer, A.D., and Feiguine, R.J. Clinical effects of amitriptyline in adolescent depression: A pilot study. *Journal of American Academy of Child Psychiatry*, 1981, **20**, 638-644.

Kranzler, G. *You can change how you feel.* Eugene, Oregon: RETC Press, 1974.

Lehmann, L. The relationship of depression to other DSM-III Axis I disorders. In E.E. Beckman and W.R. Leber (Eds.), *Handbook of depression: Treatment, assessment, and research* (pp. 669-699). Homewood, Illinois: Dorsey Press, 1985.

Lewinsohn, P.M., Antonuccio, D.O., Steinmetz-Breckenridge, J.L., and Teri, L. *The Coping with Depression Course: A psychoeducational intervention for unipolar depression.* Eugene, Oregon: Castalia Publishing Company, 1984.

Lewinsohn, P.M., and Atwood, G. Depression: A clinical-research approach. The case of MRSG. *Psychotherapy: Theory, Research, and Practice*, 1969, **6**, 166-171.

Lewinsohn, P.M., Biglan, T., and Zeiss, A. Behavioral treatment of depression. In P. Davidson (Ed.), *Behavioral management of anxiety, depression, and pain.* (pp. 91-146). New York: Brunner/Mazel, 1976.

Lewinsohn, P.M., Clarke, G.N., and Hops, H. *Cognitive-behavioral group treatment of depression in adolescents: A replication.* Unpublished manuscript, Oregon Research Institute, 1990.

Lewinsohn, P.M., Clarke, G.N., Hops, H., Andrews, J., and Osteen, V. *Cognitive-behavioral group treatment of depression in adolescents.* Paper presented at the annual meeting of the Association for Advancement of Behavior Therapy, Boston, Mass., (November) 1987.

Lewinsohn, P.M., Clarke, G.N., Hops, H., Andrews, J., and Williams, J. *Cognitive-behavioral treatment for depressed adolescents.* Unpublished manuscript, Oregon Research Institute, 1990.

Lewinsohn, P.M., Fenn, D.J., Stanton, A., and Franklin, J. The relation of age of onset to duration of episode in unipolar depression. *Journal of Psychology and Age*, 1986, **1**, 63-68.

Lewinsohn, P.M., and Graf, M. Pleasant activities and depression. *Journal of Consulting and Clinical Psychology*, 1973, **41**, 261-268.

Lewinsohn, P.M., Hoberman, H.M., and Clarke, G.N. The Coping with Depression Course: Review and future directions. *Canadian Journal of Behavioural Science*, 1989, **21**(4), 470-493.

Lewinsohn, P.M., Hoberman, H.M., and Rosenbaum, M. A prospective study of risk factors for unipolar depression. *Journal of Abnormal Psychology*, 1988, **97**(3), 251-264.

Lewinsohn, P.M., Hoberman, H.M., Teri, L., and Hautzinger, M. An integrative theory of unipolar depression. In S. Reiss, and R.R. Bootzin (Eds.), *Theoretical issues in behavioral therapy* (pp. 313-359). New York: Academic Press, 1985.

Lewinsohn, P.M., Hops, H., Roberts, R. and Seeley, J. *Adolescent depression: Prevalence and psychosocial aspects.* Boston, Mass.: Paper presented at the annual meeting of the American Public Health Association, (November) 1988.

Lewinsohn, P.M., Hops, H., Roberts, R. and Seeley, J. *The prevalence of affective and major disorders among older adolescents.* Unpublished manuscript, Oregon Research Institute, 1989.

Lewinsohn, P.M., Mermelstein, R.M., Alexander, C., and MacPhillamy, D.J. The unpleasant events schedule: A scale for the measurement of aversive events. *Journal of Clinical Psychology,* 1985, **41**, 483-498.

Lewinsohn, P.M., Mischel, W., Chaplin, W., and Barton, R. Social competence and depression: The role of illusory self-perceptions. *Journal of Abnormal Psychology*, 1980, **89**(2), 203-212.

Lewinsohn, P.M., Muñoz, R.F., Youngren, M.A., and Zeiss, A.M. *Control your depression* (revised edition). Englewood Cliffs, New Jersey: Prentice-Hall, 1986.

Lewinsohn, P.M., and Rohde, P. Psychological measurement of depression: Overview and conclusions. In A.J. Marsella, R.M.A. Hirshfeld, and M. Katz (Eds.), *The measurement of depression.* New York: Guilford Press, 1987.

Lewinsohn, P.M., and Rohde, P., Hops, H., and Clarke, G. *Leader's manual for parent groups: Adolescent Coping with Depression Course.* Eugene, Oregon: Castalia Publishing Company, 1990.

Lewinsohn, P.M., and Shaffer, M. Use of home observation as an integral part of treatment of depression: Preliminary report and case studies. *Journal of Consulting and Clinical Psychology*, 1971, **37**, 87-94.

Lewinsohn, P.M., and Shaw, D. Feedback about interpersonal behavior as an agent of behavior change: A case study in the treatment of depression. *Psychotherapy and Psychosomatics*, 1969, **17**, 82-88.

Lewinsohn, P.M., and Talkington, J. Studies on the measurement of unpleasant events and relations with depression. *Applied Psychological Measurement*, 1979, **3**, 83-101.

References

Lewinsohn, P.M., Weinstein, M., and Alper, T. A behavioral approach to the group treatment of depressed persons: A methodological contribution. *Journal of Clinical Psychology*, 1970, **26**, 525-532.

Lewinsohn, P.M., Weinstein, M., and Shaw, D. Depression: A clinical research approach. In R.D. Rubin and C.M. Frank (Eds.), *Advances in behavior therapy*. New York: Academic Press, 1969.

Lewinsohn, P.M., Youngren, M.A., and Grosscup, S.J. Reinforcement and depression. In R.A. Depue (Ed.), *The psychobiology of the depressive disorders: Implications for the effects of stress* (pp. 291-316). New York: Academic Press, 1979.

MacPhillamy, D.J., and Lewinsohn, P.M. The pleasant events schedule: Studies on reliability, validity, and scale intercorrelation. *Journal of Consulting and Clinical Psychology*, 1982, **50**, 363-380.

Manson, S.M. American Indian and Alaska native mental health research. *Journal of the National Center*, 1988, **1**(3), 1-64.

Manson, S., Mosely, R.M., and Brenneman, D.L. *Physical illness, depression, and older American Indians: A preventive intervention trial*. Unpublished manuscript, Oregon Health Sciences University, 1988.

Maser, J.D., and Clonniger, C.R. *Co-morbidity in anxiety and mood disorders*. Washington, D.C.: American Psychiatric Press, 1989.

McKnight, D.L., Nelson, R.O., Hayes, S.C., and Jarrett, R.B. Importance of treating individually-assessed response classes in the amelioration of depression. *Behavior Therapy*, 1984, **15**, 315-355.

McLean, P.D., and Carr, S. The psychological treatment of unipolar depression: Progress and limitations. *Canadian Journal of Behavioral Science*, 1989, **21**(4), 452-469.

McLean, P.D., and Hakstian, A.R. Clinical depression: Comparative efficacy of outpatient treatments. *Journal of Clinical and Counseling Psychology*, 1979, **47**(5), 818-836.

McLean, P.D., Ogston, K., and Grauer, L. A behavioral approach to the treatment of depression. *Journal of Behavioral Therapy and Experimental Psychiatry*, 1973, **4**, 323-330.

Moos, R. *Family Environment Scale and preliminary manual.* Palo Alto, California: Consulting Psychologists Press, 1974.

Muñoz R.F., and Lewinsohn, P.M. *Personal Beliefs Inventory.* Unpublished manuscript, University of Oregon, 1976.

Muñoz, R.F., Ying, Y.W., Armas, R., Chan, F., and Gurza, R. The San Francisco Depression Research Project: A randomized trial with medical outpatients. In R.F. Muñoz (Ed.), *Depression prevention: Research direction* (pp 199-215). Washington, D.C.: Hemisphere Press, 1987.

Muñoz, R.F., Ying, Y., Bernal, G., Perez-Stable, E.J., Sorensen, J.L., and Hargreaves, W.A. *The prevention of clinical depression: A randomized controlled trial.* Unpublished manuscript, University of California at San Francisco, 1988.

Murphy, G.E., Simons, A.D., Wetzel, R.D., and Lustman, P.J. Cognitive therapy and pharmacotherapy: Singly and together in the treatment of depression. *Archives of General Psychiatry*, 1984, **41**, 33-41.

Nolen-Hoeksma, S., Seligman, E.P., and Girgus, J.S. Learned helplessness in children: A longitudinal study of depression, achievement, and explanatory style. *Journal of Personality and Social Psychology.* 1986, **51**(2).

Orvaschel, H., and Puig-Antich, J. *Schedule for Affective Disorder and Schizophrenia for school-age children, Epidemiologic version: Kiddie-SADS-E (K-SADS-E) (4th version).* Technical report, Western Psychiatric Institute and Clinic, Pittsburgh, Penn., 1986

Paykel, E.S., Myers, J.K., Dienelt, M.N., Klerman, G.L., Lindenthal, J.J., and Pepper, M.P. Life events and depression. *Archives of General Psychiatry*, 1969, **21**, 753-760.

Petti, T.A., Bornstein, M., Delemater, A., and Conners, C.K. Evaluation and multimodality treatment of a depressed prepubertal girl. *Journal of the American Academy of Child Psychiatry*, 1980, **19**, 690-702.

References

Pfeffer, C.R. *The suicidal child*. New York: Guilford Press, 1986.

Preskorn, S.H., Weller, E.B., and Weller, R.A. Depression in children: Relationship between plasma imipramine levels and response. *Journal of Clinical Psychiatry*, 1982, **43**, 450-453.

Puig-Antich, J., Lukens, E., Davies, M., Goetz, D., Brennan-Quattrock, J., and Todak, G. Psychosocial functioning in prepubertal major depressive disorders: I. Interpersonal relationships during the depressive episode. *Archives of General Psychiatry*, 1985, **42**, 500-507.

Puig-Antich, J., Perel, J.M., Lupatkin, W., Chambers, W.J., Tabrizi, M.A., King, J., Goetz, R., Davies, M., and Stiller, R.L. Imipramine in prepubertal major depressive disorders. *Archives of General Psychiatry*, 1987, **44**, 81-89.

Radloff, L.S. A CES-D scale: A self-report depression scale for research in the general population. *Applied Psychological Measurement*, 1977, **1**, 385-401.

Rancurello, M. Clinical applications of antidepressant drugs in childhood: Behavioral and emotional disorders. *Psychiatric Annals*, 1985, **15**, 88-100.

Rehm, L.P. A self-control model of depression. *Behavior Therapy*, 1977, **8**, 787-804.

Reynolds, W.M. *Suicidal Ideation Questionnaire*. Odessa, Florida: Psychological Assessment Resources, 1987.

Reynolds, W.M., and Coats, K.I. A comparison of cognitive-behavioral therapy and relaxation training for the treatment of depression in adolescents. *Journal of Consulting and Clinical Psychology*, 1986, **54**, 653-660.

Roberts, R., Andrews, J., Lewinsohn, P.M., and Hops, H. Assessment of depression in adolescents using the Center for Epidemiological Studies—Depression Scale (CES-D). *Journal of Consulting and Clinical Psychology*, in press.

Roberts, R.E., Lewinsohn, P.M., and Seeley, J.R. *Screening for Adolescent Depression: A comparison of the CES-D and BDI.* Manuscript submitted for publication, 1990.

Robin, A.L. An approach to teaching parents and adolescents problem-solving communication skills: A preliminary report. *Behavior Therapy*, 1977, **8**, 639-643.

Robin, A.L. Problem-solving communication training: A behavioral approach to the treatment of parent-adolescent conflict. *The American Journal of Family Therapy*, 1979, **7**, 69-82.

Robin, A.L. A controlled evaluation of problem-solving communication training with parent adolescent conflict. *Behavior Therapy*, 1981, **12**, 593-609.

Robin, A.L., Kent, R.N., O'Leary, K.D., Foster, S., and Prinz, R.J. An approach to teaching parents and adolescents problem-solving communication skills: A preliminary report. *Behavior Therapy*, 1977, **8**, 639-643.

Robin, A.L., and Weiss, J.G. Criterion-related validity of behavioral and self-report measures of problem-solving communication skills in distressed and nondistressed parent-adolescent dyads. *Behavioral Assessment*, 1980, **3**, 339-352.

Robinson, J.C., and Lewinsohn, P.M. Behavior modification of speech characteristics in a chronically depressed man. *Behavior Therapy*, 1973, **4**, 150-152.

Rosenbaum, M. Individual differences in self-control behaviors and tolerance of painful stimulation. *Journal of Abnormal Psychology*, 1980, **89**(4), 581-590.

Rosenberg, M. Rosenberg Self-Esteem Scale. In M. Rosenberg, *Conceiving the Self* (pp. 201-205). New York: Basic Books, 1979.

Rotheram, M.J. Evaluation of imminent danger for suicide among youth. *American Journal of Orthopsychiatry*, 1987, **57**, 102-160.

References

Rude, S.S., and Rehm, L.P. *Cognitive and behavioral predictors of response to treatments for depression.* Unpublished manuscript, 1989.

Rush, A.J., Beck, A.T., Kovacs, M., and Hollon, S. Comparative efficacy of cognitive therapy and pharmacotherapy in the treatment of depressed outpatients. *Cognitive Therapy and Research*, 1977, **1**(1), 17-37.

Ryan, N.D., Puig-Antich, J., Cooper, T., Rabinovich, H., Ambrosini, P., Davies, M., King, J., Torres, D., and Fried, J. Imipramine in adolescent major depression: Plasma level and clinical response. *Acta Psychiatrica Scandinavica*, 1985, **73**, 275-288.

Sacco, W.P., and Beck, A.T. Cognitive therapy of depression. In E.E. Beckman and W.R. Leber (Eds.), *Handbook of depression: Treatment, assessment, and research* (pp. 3-38). Homewood, Illinois: Dorsey Press, 1985.

Sanchez, V.C., Lewinsohn, P.M., and Larson, D.W. Assertion training: Effectiveness in the treatment of depression. *Journal of Clinical Psychology*, 1980, **36**, 526-529.

Sandler, I.N., and Block, M. Life stress and maladaption of children. *American Journal of Community Psychology*, 1979, **1**, 425-440.

Schulberg, H.C., McClelland, M., and Burns, B.J. Depression and physical illness: The prevalence, causation, and diagnosis of co-morbidity. *Clinical Psychology Review*, 1987, **7**, 145-167.

Seligman, M.E.P., Peterson, C., Kaslow, N.J., Tanenbaum, R.L., Alloy, L.B., and Abramson, L.Y. Attributional style and depressive symptoms among children. *Journal of Abnormal Psychology*, 1984, **93**, 242-247.

Shaffer, D., and Fisher, P. The epidemiology of suicide in children and young adolescents. *Journal of the American Academy of Child Psychiatry*, 1981, **20**, 545-565.

Simeon, J.G., Ferguson, H.B., Copping, W.M., and DiNicola, V.F. *Fluoxetine effect in adolescent depression.* Seattle, Washington: Paper presented at the annual meeting of the American Academy of Child and Adolescent Depression, (October) 1988.

Simons, A.D., Garfield, S.L., and Murphy, G.E. The process of change in cognitive therapy and pharmacotherapy for depression: Changes in mood and cognition. *Archives of General Psychiatry*, 1984, **41**, 45-51.

Simons, A.D., Lustman, P.J., Wetzel, R.D., and Murphy, G.E. Predicting response to cognitive therapy of depression: The role of learned resourcefulness. *Cognitive Therapy and Research*, 1985, **9**, 79-89.

Spitzer, R.L., and Endicott, J. *Schedule for Affective Disorders and Schizophrenia—Change Version* (SADS-C). New York State Psychiatric Institute, 1978.

Spitzer, R.L., Endicott, J., and Robins, E. Research diagnostic criteria: Rationale and reliability. *Archives of General Psychiatry*, 1978, **35**, 773-782.

Steinbrueck, S.M., Maxwell, S.E., and Howard, G.S. A meta-analysis of psychotherapy and drug therapy in the treatment of unipolar depression with adults. *Journal of Consulting and Clinical Psychology*, 1983, **51**, 856-863.

Steinmetz, J.L., Breckenridge, J.R., Thompson, L.W., and Gallagher, D. Some predictors of successful treatment for elderly depressives. Paper presented in L. Thompson (Chair), *Treatment of major depression in older adults: First year results.* Anaheim, California: A symposium presented at the annual meeting of the American Psychological Association, (August) 1983.

Steinmetz, J.L., Lewinsohn, P.M., and Antonuccio, D.O. Prediction of individual outcome in a group intervention for depression. *Journal of Consulting and Clinical Psychology*, 1983, **51**, 331-337.

Strauss, C.C., Forehand, R., Frame, C., and Smith, K. Characteristics of children with extreme scores on the children's depression inventory. *Journal of Consulting and Clinical Psychology*, 1984, **13**, 227-231.

Teri, L., and Lewinsohn, P.M. Group intervention for unipolar depression. *The Behavior Therapist*, 1985, **8**, 109-111.

Trautman, P., and Shaffer, D. Treatment of child and adolescent suicide attempters. In H. Sudak, A. Ford, and N. Rushforth (Eds.), *Suicide in the young.* Boston, Mass.: John Wright PSG, 1984.

References

Turner, R.W., Wehl, C.K., Cannon, D.S., and Craig, K.A. *Individual treatment for depression in alcoholics: A comparison of behavioral, cognitive, and nonspecific therapy.* VA Medical Center, Salt Lake City, unpublished mimeograph, 1980.

Weissman, A.N., and Beck, A.T. *Development and validation of the dysfunctional attitude scale.* Paper presented a the annual meeting of the Association for the Advancement of Behavior Therapy, Chicago, Illinois, 1978.

Weissman, M.M., Gammon, D., John, K., Merikangas, K.R., Warner, V., Prussoff, B.A., and Sholomskas, D. Children of depressed parents: Increased psychopathology and early onset of major depression. *Archives of General Psychiatry*, 1987, **44**, 847-853.

Weissman, M.M., and Klerman, G.L. The chronic depressive in the community: Unrecognized and poorly treated. *Comprehensive Psychiatry*, 1977, **18**, 523-532.

Weissman, M.M., Klerman, G.L., Prusoff, B.A., Sholomskas, D., and Padin, N. Depressed outpatients one year after treatment with drugs and/or interpersonal therapy. *Archives of General Psychiatry*, 1981, **38**, 51-55.

Weissman, M.M., Orvaschel, H., and Padian, N. Children's symptom and social functioning self-report scales: Comparison of mothers' and children's reports. *Journal of Nervous and Mental Disease*, 1980, **168**, 736-740.

Weissman, M.M., and Paykel, E.S. *The depressed woman.* Chicago: University of Chicago Press, 1974.

Weissman, M.M., Prusoff, B.A., DiMascio, A., Neu, C., Goklaney, M., and Klerman, G.L. The efficacy of drugs and psychotherapy in the treatment of acute depressive episodes. *American Journal of Psychiatry*, 1979, **136**, 555-558.

Yalom, I.D. *The theory and practice of group psychotherapy.* New York: Basic Books, 1970.

Youngren, M.A., and Lewinsohn, P.M. The functional relation between depression and problematic interpersonal behavior. *Journal of Abnormal Psychology*, 1980, **89**, 333-341.

Zeiss, A.M., Lewinsohn, P.M., and Muñoz, R.F. Nonspecific improvement effects in depression using interpersonal, cognitive, and pleasant events focused treatments. *Journal of Consulting and Clinical Psychology*, 1979, **47**, 427-439.